Aids to Undergraduate Surgery

Simon Loughe
Darwin College
Cambridge

DEDICATION

To my mother and father.

Aids to Undergraduate Surgery

Peter M. Mowschenson

BSc., M.B., B.S., M.R.C.P., F.R.C.S.
Senior Registrar in Surgery and Honorary Lecturer
Guys Hospital and University of London
Clinical Fellow and Chief Resident in Surgery
Harvard Medical School and Beth Israel Hospital
Boston, Massachusetts

CHURCHILL LIVINGSTONE
EDINBURGH LONDON AND NEW YORK 1978

CHURCHILL LIVINGSTONE
Medical Division of Longman Group Limited

Distributed in the United States of America by
Churchill Livingstone Inc., 19 West 44th Street,
New York, N.Y. 10036 and by associated companies,
branches and representatives throughout
the world.

First Edition 1978
  Reprinted 1979
  Reprinted 1981

ISBN 0 443 01328 4

British Library Cataloguing in Publication Data

Mowschenson, Peter M
  Aids to undergraduate surgery.
  1. Preoperative care   2. Postoperative care
  I. Title
617'.919   RD51   77-30529

Printed in Singapore by
Singapore Offset Printing Pte Ltd

Preface

The purpose of this book is to help the reader review information he has already acquired from comprehensive sources, and also provide a stimulus for further reading.

The nature of the text leaves little room for discussion, and this could be misleading if the text is used as a main source of information. Where numbers are given these are approximate and do not give the full range.

I thank the surgeons and physicians at Beth Israel, Guy's and Salem hospitals who gave me helpful criticism.

I am indebted to Sharyn Brooks for her excellent secretarial assistance.

I also thank Moon.

Boston 1978   P.M.M.

Contents

Fluid and electrolytes

ANATOMY OF BODY WATER

70 kg man (ml)		% of body weight
3500	Plasma	5%
10500	Interstitial fluid	15%
28000	Intracellular fluid	40%
42000	Total body water	60% for males
		50% for females

APPROXIMATE VOLUME AND ELECTROLYTE CONTENT OF GASTROINTESTINAL FLUIDS

	Volume (ml)	Na	K	Cl	HCO_3 (mmol/l)
Gastric	1500–2000	60	10	120	0–25
Pancreatic	500–1000	140	5	75	80
Bile	300–1000	148	5	100	35
Small bowel	1000–3000	110	5	100	30
Diarrhoea	500–17000	120	25	90	45

SODIUM BALANCE

Predominant extracellular cation. Normal diet: 50-90 mmol/day. With normal kidneys, urine loss can be less than 1 mmol/day, in face of salt restriction.

Causes of hyponatraemia
1. Water overload—iatrogenic
2. Head injuries—inappropriate ADH release
3. Addison's disease

Complications
Convulsions

Treatment
1. Water restriction
2. Steroids for Addison's

Causes of hypernatraemia
Water deprivation

Complications
1. Delirium
2. Hyperthermia
3. Oliguria

Treatment
Rehydrate

POTASSIUM BALANCE

Predominant intracellular cation. Normal diet 50-100 mmol/day
Urine excretion related to distal tubular exchange with Na^+ and H^+
Daily replacement: about 80 mmol.

Causes of hyperkalaemia
1. Renal failure
2. Trauma
3. Acidosis

↑ K⊕ a) RF
b) trauma
c) acidosis
⇓
heart block
cardiac arrest

Complications
1. Heart block
2. Diastolic arrest

Treatment of hyperkalaemia
1. Immediate: 80 mmol Na lactate/bicarbonate
2. 100 ml 50% dextrose with 10 units insulin i.v.
3. Cation exchange resin
4. Dialysis

Causes of hypokalaemia
1. Excess renal loss
   (i)   Diuretics
   (ii) Hyperaldosteronism
   (iii) Cushing's disease
2. Gastrointestinal losses
   (i)   Diarrhoea
   (ii) Vomiting (mainly renal loss)
   (iii) Fistulae

↓ K⊕ renal
a) diuretics
b) Hyperaldosterone
c) Cushings
GI
diarrhoea
vomiting
Fistulae
⇓
weakness
ileus
arrhythmias
digitalis sensitivity

Complications
1. Muscle weakness and extreme lethargy
2. Ileus
3. Cardiac arrhythmias
4. Digitalis sensitivity

Treatment
1. Prevent: adequate daily replacement
2. Not more than 30 mmol/hr. Concentrated solutions via central
   line to avoid phlebitis

CALCIUM $[Ca^{2\oplus}]$
Mostly stored in bone
Diet 1–3 g/day
Urine excretion less than 300 mg/day. Remainder in faeces

Causes of hypocalcaemia
1. Following surgery for hyperparathyroidism or thyroidectomy
2. Acute pancreatitis → *chelated*
3. Hypoparathyroidism → *↓ parathormone*
4. Malabsorption syndromes → *↓ intake*
5. Pancreatic and small bowel fistulae → *↑ losses*
6. Massive soft tissue infections →
7. Severe magnesium depletion →

Complications
1. Tetany
2. Convulsions

Rx = IV. calcium gluconate

Treatment of tetany
10 ml of 10% calcium gluconate i.v. as a bolus and repeat as
necessary

Hypercalcaemia
See Hyperparathyroidism, p. 33.

MAGNESIUM BALANCE $[Mg^{2\oplus}]$
50% in bone
Diet: 240 mg/day
Excretion mostly in stool, some in urine
Serum level is not a true reflection of body magnesium

Causes of magnesium deficiency
↓Mg → starved
1. Starvation   *malabsorbed*
2. Malabsorption   *↑ GI. fluid loss*
3. Protracted gastrointestinal fluid loss   *pancreatitis*
4. Pancreatitis   *Conn's Syn.*
5. Conn's syndrome   *alcoholism*
6. Chronic alcoholism   *burns*
7. Burns   *IV. Rx č Mg supplements*
8. Prolonged i.v. infusion without magnesium supplements

Complications
Similar to hypocalcaemia   *tetany & convulsions*

Treatment

Prevent. Give 1.2g MgSO₄ (equivalent to 240mg Mg) i.v./day to
patients liable to become deficient

IV. MgSO₄

Causes of magnesium excess
1. Chronic renal failure
2. Excess antacid therapy with Mg salts in patients with renal failure

Complications
ECG changes of hyperkalaemia

Treatment
Correct acidosis and volume depletion

[handwritten: ↑Mg a) CRF b) Xses antacid Rx + RF]

[handwritten: ↑K⊕ ECG △]

[handwritten: Rx = anted acidosis & vol, deplet.]

WATER BALANCE
(Adults)

Intake
Oral—2000–2500 ml
Metabolic—200 ml   *[handwritten: 3 lt/day]*

Output

Sensible
- Urine — 800–1500 ml
- Stool — 200 ml
- Sweat — 0–4000 ml/hr depending on temperature elevat

Insensible
- Lungs
- Skin
12 ml/kg/24 hrs.

Concept of third space loss
Translocation of extracellular fluid into peritoneum, bowel, tissues, etc., following trauma e.g., surgery, sepsis, inflammation. Fluid remains extra-cellular, but is 'lost,' since it does not participate in normal exchange with other fluid compartments

EVALUATION OF PATIENT'S FLUID AND ELECTROLYTE REQUIREMENTS
1. Examine patient
2. Review previous input and output
3. Note patient's weight—patients normally lose ¼ to ½ lb/day on i.v. fluids

Replace
1. Measured losses
   (i) Gastrointestinal with normal saline
   (ii) Urine output with 5% dextrose
   Normal urine volume 1000 ml/day.
2. Insensible loss
   (i) 12 ml/kg/24 h with 5% dextrose
   (ii) plus extra for fever
3. Predict third space losses—depends on type of surgery/disease—replace with saline
4. Potassium—give 60 mmol/day basic requirement +30-40 mmol/1 of normal saline for gastrointestinal losses to prevent alkalosis and hypokalaemia

In general, by careful recording of input and output and careful daily weights, serum electrolyte determinations are only required if indicated. Fluid orders are best written for fixed 24-hour periods e.g., 8:00 AM-8:00 AM, except for patients with large volume changes where frequent review is necessary

PARENTERAL FEEDING
The vast majority of patients undergoing surgery have normal energy reserves, and can withstand the period of catabolism without intravenous calories

Indications for parenteral feeding   TPN
1. Patients with severe malnutrition requiring major surgery. e.g., malignant disease, oesophageal stricture
2. Patients with postoperative complications leading to delayed return of oral feeding e.g., prolonged ileus, enteric fistulae
3. Patients with prolonged sepsis and renal failure who are severely catabolic
4. Patients with short bowel syndrome following extensive resection

Complications of parenteral feeding
1. Pneumothorax, haemothorax, cardiac tamponade—during insertion of central line
2. Sepsis—solution, line, catheter (bacterial/fungal)
3. Metabolic changes:
   (i) Hyperosmolar states
   (ii) Hypo/hypernatraemia
   (iii) Hypophosphataemia
   (iv) Calcium/magnesium abnormalities
   (v) Fatty acid deficiency
   (vi) Reactive hypoglycaemia—if solution stops running suddenly
   (vii) Hyperammonaemia
   (viii) Acidosis

Shock   Hypovolaemic / Septic / Cardiogenic

Shock results when tissue/organ blood flow is inadequate to maintain normal cellular activity. Usually accompanied by hypotension, oliguria, cutaneous vasoconstriction

TRAUMATIC SHOCK
Internal/External bleeding

Pathophysiology
Blood loss→diminished blood volume→diminished venous return, fall in cardiac output and blood pressure. Baroreceptor stimulation→ sympatho adrenal response→decrease in regional blood flow through splanchnic, renal, pulmonary, cutaneous area (α receptor areas). Constriction affects precapillary arterioles and postcapillary venules. Capillary hydrostatic pressure drop leads to net inflow of extravascular fluid, tending to compensate blood loss. In cases of severe blood loss persistent vasoconstriction results in accumulation of anaerobic metabolic products e.g., lactate. Precapillary arterioles relax, but postcapillary venules remain constricted. (Mechanism unknown). Capillary hydrostatic pressure increase leads to net loss of fluid from vascular compartment and stagnant hypoxia tending to potentiate blood loss. Marks stage of irreversible shock. Red and white cells aggregate in stagnant capillaries forming microthrombi and disseminated intravascular coagulation (DIC) is initiated

SEPTIC SHOCK
With increased use of antibiotics gram negative organisms are evolving as most common cause:

Sites of origin
1. Urinary tract
   (i) pyelonephritis
   (ii) catheterization
   (iii) instrumentation
2. Pneumonias
3. Wound infections
4. Abscesses e.g., subphrenic (E. coli, klebsiella, proteus, pseudomonas, bacteroides)

Pathophysiology:

1. *Circulating lipopolysaccharide Endotoxin.* Released from walls of dead bacteria combines with antibody and complement to form anaphylotoxin. →Release of vasoactive substances e.g., catecholamines, histamine. Causes pooling of blood chiefly in splanchnic bed, lungs→diminished venous return and baroreceptor stimulation. Persistent stimulation leads to stagnant hypoxia as with blood loss

2. *Living Bacteria.* Interact with damaged tissues to release kinins. Causes A-V shunting which decreases total peripheral resistance and leads to high cardiac output. Shunting potentiates ischaemia in areas of stagnant hypoxia i.e., high cardiac output is accompanied by decreased O_2 delivery to tissues and decrease *paradox* A-V O_2 difference

CARDIOGENIC SHOCK

1. Postmyocardial infarction
2. Post heart surgery

Pathophysiology:
Decreased myocardial contractility→decreased cardiac output and baroreceptor stimulation→ Increased total peripheral resistance→increase in left ventricular after load→potentiation of myocardial ischaemia and further impairment of contractility. Persistent vasoconstriction leads to stagnant hypoxia

CHANGES IN CELL METABOLISM IN SHOCK

1. Lactic acid accumulation—anaerobic metabolism
2. Decrease in ATP production—anaerobic metabolism
3. Membrane function
   (i) Sodium leaks into cells. Potassium leaks out of cells
   (ii) Lyosomes fragment→autodigestion
4. Fatty acid mobilisation
   (i) Ketonaemia
   (ii) Fat emboli to lung—controversial

SPECIFIC ORGAN FAILURE

1. Kidneys—acute tubular necrosis
2. Lungs—adult respiratory distress syndrome
3. Gut—nonocclusive infarction

HIGH RISK PATIENTS

Traumatic Shock. Fractures e.g., pelvis, GI bleeding, postoperative bleeding   RTAs

Septic Shock. Urinary tract and bowel surgery, burns, immunosuppressants, steroids, diabetes

Cardiogenic Shock. Elderly, previous myocardial infarction

TREATMENT OF SHOCK

1. Prevent—identify high risk patients early
2. Diagnosis of underlying cause
3. Correction of hypovolaemia—guided by CVP, or more accurately, pulmonary capillary wedge pressure with Swan Ganz catheter, hourly urine output, haematocrit
4. Correction of acid/base/electrolytes e.g., bicarbonate for acidosis
5. Antibiotics: Septic shock. After cultures give broad spectrum drugs. e.g., ampicillin and gentamycin. If anaerobes e.g., bacteroides thought to be present add clindamycin/chloramphenicol/metronidazole
6. Pressors: vasoconstrictors make shock worse. In cardiogenic shock stimulation of contractility e.g., with dopamine/isoprenalin can increase cardiac output measured with Swan Ganz catheter
7. Steroids: massive doses e.g., 30 mg prednisone/kg—very controversial
8. Vasodilators: e.g., phenoxybenzamine, chlorpromazine—controversial
9. Antacids: may prevent stress ulcers
10. Surgery
    (i)   Stop bleeding
    (ii)   Drain pus
    (iii) Remove dead bowel
    (iv)   Intra-aortic balloon pump for cardiogenic shock
11. Ventilation for pulmonary failure. Positive end expiratory pressure is particularly important
12. Dialysis for renal failure
13. Heparin for DIC

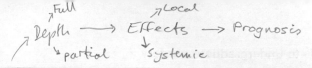

Robbie **Burns**

DEPTH OF BURN
1. Partial thickness—healing can occur from epithelial remnants
2. Full thickness—total destruction of all epithelial remnants.

LOCAL EFFECTS OF BURN
1. Pain
2. Loss of fluid, electrolytes, protein
3. Heat loss—increased calorie requirement
4. Infection—staphylococcal initially
   —gram negatives especially pseudomonas after 5 days
   —streptococci can convert partial thickness burns to full thickness
5. Thrombosis
   (i) From heat
   (ii) In electrical burns

SYSTEMIC EFFECTS OF BURN
1. Haemolysis
   (i) direct effect of heat
   (ii) increased red cell fragility
2. Generalised increase in capillary permeability. With exudation of fluid into ECF and wound
3. Salt and water loss—50% of plasma volume can be lost within 3 hours in 40% burn
4. Diminished cardiac output
   (i) Direct effect of circulating toxic substances
   (ii) Increased blood viscosity and peripheral resistance
5. Oliguria and renal failure
   (i) Hypovolaemia
   (ii) Haemoglobinuria
   (iii) Proteinuria
6. Curling's ulcer—may be related to disruption of mucosal barrier
7. Respiratory failure
   (i) Sepsis
   (ii) Fluid overload
   (iii) Inhalation of smoke and carbon monoxide
8. Catabolism
   (i) Heat loss
   (ii) Sepsis
   (iii) Complications e.g., renal/respiratory failure

PROGNOSIS
If age plus % of burn is more than 100, then mortality approaches 100%, mainly from toxaemia. Children do worse

SURFACE AREA ESTIMATION
Rule of 9's—unreliable in children (small limbs)
Head and neck 9
Each arm 9
Each leg 9 × 2
Front of trunk 9 × 2
Back of trunk 9 × 2   = 73%
Perineum 1

General management of burns
1. Sedation and analgesia: Requirement inversely proportional to depth of burn
2. Ensure adequate airway
3. Fluid balance: Formulae are only a guide to initial management. Modify according to response
    (i)   Hourly urine output, greater than ½ml/kg/hr
    (ii) CVP
    (iii) Haematocrit
    (iv) Electrolytes and acid base status

    Formula for first 24 hours
    (i)   1ml/% burn/kg/day of Ringer's soln. ⎤ up to 50%
          1ml/% burn/kg/day of Plasma/Dextran ⎦ in adults
    (ii) Maintenance fluids in addition
    (iii) For next 24hrs give half the amount for the burn in addition to normal maintenance
          In children specially prepared tables should be used
4. Blood as necessary
5. Tetanus prophylaxis
6. Five day course of penicillin vs. streptococci
7. Antacids—may prevent Curling's ulcer
8. Nutrition; Give orally whenever possible
9. Psychological aspects. Extremely important. Requires great efforts by all involved in patient care
10. Rehabilitation

Local burn care.
Much depends on personal preference and policy of different burn units. The open method tends to be used on large areas which are difficult to dress; the closed method for smaller burns and for burns of the extremities. The different methods may include:

(i)   Debridement; using saline soaked dressings or direct removal of necrotic material. Latter is often best carried out in operating theatre

(ii)   Prevention of infection—Topical agents (e.g. silver sulphadiazine) are applied to the burn. Isolation beds, laminar flow, and sterile dressing techniques are complimentary

(iii) Homografts. These may be used as a temporary dressing. They render the underlying tissues sterile in 24hrs, and also reduce fluid loss

(iv)   Autografts. Areas of full thickness loss which have been rendered suitable as recipient sites by debridement or homografts are grafted

(v)   Escharotomy. Circumferential extremity burns may impede circulation. Doppler may be used to detect a distal pulse. If elevation fails to restore distal pulse then the eschar is cut. No anaesthetic is required

(vi)   Maintenance of function:
       Eye burns, Protect cornea
       Prevent limb contractures

Malignant disease in general

MORTALITY FROM CANCER (IN DECREASING FREQUENCY)

Men	Women
Lung	Breast
Colon/rectum	Colon/rectum
Stomach	Uterus
Prostate	Lung
Pancreas	Ovary

AETIOLOGY OF MALIGNANT DISEASE
1. Chemical e.g.,
    (i) Smoking—lung cancer
    (ii) Asbestos—mesothelioma
    (iii) ß-naphthylamine—urinary tract
2. Physical e.g.,
    (i) X-rays—leukaemia
    (ii) Ultraviolet light—skin cancer
3. Viral e.g.,
    EB virus—Burkitt's lymphoma
4. Genetic e.g.,
    Familial polyposis coli
5. Miscellaneous
    Geographical, diet

SPREAD OF MALIGNANT DISEASE
1. Direct extension e.g., longitudinal growth of oesophageal cancer
2. Lymphatic e.g., especially carcinomas
3. Vascular e.g., especially sarcomas and carcinomas
4. Transcoelomic e.g., stomach

CLINICAL MANIFESTATIONS OF MALIGNANT DISEASE

1. **Effect of primary tumour**
   (i) Expansive growth e.g., obstruction, lump
   (ii) Infiltrative growth e.g., pain from nerve involvement, fixation of tumour
   (iii) Necrosis—bleeding/infection

2. **Effect of metastases**
   (i) Lymphadenopathy
   (ii) Lung secondaries (dyspnoea)
   (iii) Liver secondaries (jaundice)
   (iv) Bone secondaries (fractures)
   (v) Brain secondaries (epilepsy)
   (vi) Skin secondaries (nodules)

3. **Systemic manifestations of malignant disease**
   (i) Cachexia, weight loss, anaemia, fever
   (ii) Cutaneous e.g., acanthosis nigricans (lung, stomach), dermatomyositis
   (iii) Haematological e.g., polycythaemia (kidney/cerebellum)
   (iv) Vascular e.g., thrombophlebitis (lung, pancreas)
   (v) Hormonal and metabolic e.g.,
       Cushing's (lung)
       ADH secretion (lung)
       hypercalcaemia (lung-breast)
       hypoglycaemia (liver)
   (vi) Gout e.g., lymphomas
   (vii) Neuromuscular e.g.,
       cerebellar degeneration (lung)
       myasthenia gravis (thymus)

DANGER SIGNALS OF CANCER

1. Change in bowel/bladder habit
2. Nonhealing sore
3. Unusual bleeding or discharge
4. Breast lump
5. Dysphagia
6. Obvious change in wart/mole
7. Persistent cough/hoarseness

PRINCIPLES OF MANAGEMENT

1. *Diagnosis*
   (i)   History, physical examination
   (ii) Appropriate investigation
   (iii) Biopsy and staging

2. *Optimum treatment for individual patient*
   (i)   No treatment e.g., incurable elderly patient
   (ii)   Surgery alone, e.g., basal cell carcinoma
   (iii) Surgery and radiotherapy e.g., seminoma
   (iv)   Radiation alone e.g., I/II Hodgkin's
   (v)   Chemotherapy e.g., IV lymphoma
   (vi)   Radiotherapy, chemotherapy and surgery—Wilm's tumour
   (vii) Immunotherapy—under investigation

General condition of patient and associated illnesses e.g., severe congestive failure, will influence choice of treatment

TYPES OF OPERATION FOR CANCER

1. Wide local excision e.g., basal cell
2. Radical local excision e.g., melanoma
3. Radical local excision with en bloc lymph node dissection e.g., radical mastectomy
4. Extensive procedures e.g., pelvic exenteration for recurrent cervical carcinoma
5. Surgery for recurrent cancer e.g., obstruction after bowel resection
6. Resection of metastases e.g., lung/liver
7. Palliative surgery e.g., colostomy, gastrojejunostomy

Radiation therapy

Can destroy neoplastic tissue with minimal damage to surrounding tissue. i.e., good functional and cosmetic result

MECHANISM OF ACTION
Radiation causes ionisation of water in cells. Hydroxy and peroxide radicals which form cause DNA and chromosome disruption. Neoplastic cells are more sensitive
RAD is unit of measurement and expresses amount absorbed
4500–6000 rads is lethal dose for most tumours

COMPLICATIONS OF RADIOTHERAPY
1. Malaise, nausea, vomiting
2. Skin ulceration
3. Stricture, ulceration, perforation of bowel
4. Nephritis
5. Gonadal atrophy
6. Pancytopaenia
7. Pneumonitis and fibrosis
8. Pericarditis
9. Conjunctivitis/cataracts
10. Cerebral oedema/myelitis
11. Bone necrosis
12. Increased incidence of malignancy e.g., leukaemia

INDICATIONS FOR PALLIATIVE IRRADIATION
1. Pain e.g., bone secondaries
2. Haemorrhage e.g., lung cancer
3. Intractable cough e.g., lung cancer
4. Dysphagia e.g., oesophageal cancer
5. SVC obstruction e.g., carcinoma of bronchus
6. Pathologic fractures e.g., bronchus, breast
7. Spinal cord compression e.g., metastatic disease
8. Skin secondaries e.g., breast

INDICATIONS FOR PREOPERATIVE IRRADIATION
1. Carcinoma—larynx (see page 26)
2. Uterus
3. Bladder (see page 114)
4. Oesophagus—controversial (see page 58)
5. Rectum—controversial (see page 70)

Advantages of preoperative irradiation
1. Reduces bulk of tumour
2. Reduces fixation to surrounding structures
3. **May** decrease local recurrence
4. **May** increase cure rate

INDICATIONS FOR POSTOPERATIVE IRRADIATION
1. Inadequate tumour margin following resection
2. Seminoma (periaortic and iliac nodes)
3. Wilm's tumour

Complications

DIAGNOSIS OF POSTOPERATIVE FEVERS
1. History e.g.,
   (i)   Chest pain: pulmonary embolus
   (ii)   Wound pain: infection
   (iii) Arm pain: i.v. phlebitis
   (iv)   Diarrhoea: pelvic abscess
   (v)   Dysuria: urinary infection, etc.
   (vi)   Joint pain: gout
2. Physical examination e.g.,
   (i)   Wound
   (ii)   Chest
   (iii) Calf—diameter, tenderness
   (iv)   Rectal—pelvic abscess; prostatitis (catheter)
   (v)   Mouth—parotitis
   (vi)   Skin–rash—decubiti etc.
3. Review of drugs: antibiotics—allergy
4. Urine microscopy and culture
5. Chest X-ray: as indicated
6. Blood cultures
7. Other tests as indicated

PROPHYLAXIS OF DEEP VEIN THROMBOSIS
1. Early ambulation
2. Pneumatic boots, calf stimulation
3. Subcutaneous heparin (5 000 units s.c. every twelve/eight hours)
4. Aspirin
5. Oral anticoagulants
6. Intermittent Dextran 70

Diagnosis of deep vein thrombosis
1. Clinical—unreliable. Signs may be present without thrombosis and vice versa.
2. Radioiodine labelled fibrinogen—shows 30% of patients have thrombosis following surgery

Disadvantages
   (i) Not good above midthigh (most pulmonary emboli may originate above this level)
   (ii) Not good for established thrombi
   (iii) Contraindicated in pregnancy
   (iv) Incisions in lower limb can give false results
   (v) Risk of hepatitis
3. Doppler
   (i) good above mid thigh
   (ii) will not detect nonocclusive thrombus or occlusive thrombus if large collateral veins
4. Phlebography:
   (i) Any vessel
   (ii) Indicates extent and degree of fixity of thrombus

HIGH RISK FACTORS FOR PULMONARY EMBOLUS
1. Extensive trauma/surgery
2. Elderly, obese
3. Splenectomy, hip/pelvic surgery
4. Malignant disease
5. Oestrogens
6. Previous thrombosis/embolism
7. Myocardial infarction

Diagnosis of pulmonary embolus
1. History
2. Physical Examination
3. Confirm with
   (i) Blood gases 80% have decrease in pO_2
   (ii) Chest x-ray: limited value
   (iii) Lung scan: most useful
   (iv) Pulmonary arteriogram
   (v) EKG: variable changes $S_I Q_{III}$ Inverted T in III is classical

Treatment

Medical:
1. i.v. Heparin
2. Oral anticoagulation
3. Streptokinase

Surgery
1. Thrombectomy
   (i) Free-floating thrombus
   (ii) With impending venous gangrene of limb
   (iii) Massive pulmonary embolus
2. IVC Clip/plication/umbrella
   a. recurrent emboli
   b. if anticoagulation is contraindicated

CAUSES OF FAT EMBOLISM
1. Fractures e.g., tibia, hip
2. Extensive trauma
3. Burns
4. Severe infection
5. Pancreatitis
6. Closed cardiac massage

Clinical features of fat embolism
1. Dyspnoea, hypoxaemia (cyanosis)
2. Altered level of consciousness
3. Focal cerebral signs
4. Petechial haemorrhages—skin, mucosae, fundi—mainly upper half of body
5. High fever

Diagnosis of fat embolism
Physical signs develop only late
1. Earliest change is hypoxaemia
2. Chest X-ray: scattered consolidation (snow storm)
3. Fat in:
   (i) Sputum—unreliable
   (ii) Urine—in severe cases
   (iii) Blood—frozen section of whole blood stained for fat
4. Elevated lipase (exclude pancreatitis)

Management of fat embolism
1. Prevent—careful handling of fractures
2. Oxygen
3. Steroids: probably beneficial especially if given early
4. Heparin, dextran: doubtful—may potentiate intrapulmonary bleeding
5. Ventilation with positive end expiratory pressure has resulted in considerable success in severe cases

INFECTIONS

Tetanus prophylaxis
1. Meticulous debridement of devitalised tissue and foreign bodies. Do not close contaminated wounds
2. Clean wounds
    (i)   Patients without previous immunization: 0.5 ml tet. tox. followed by further dose at 6 and 12 weeks
    (ii) Previously immunised patients, but no booster within 5 years: 0.5 ml tet. tox.
3. Dirty wounds
    (i)   Patients without previous immunisation or immunised, but no booster within 5 years: 250 units of human immune globulin 0.5 ml tet. tox. followed by full course
    (ii) Previously immunised patients with booster within 12 months; no extra immunisation required
4. Antibiotics as indicated for dirty wounds

Indications for prophylactic antibiotics
1. Patients at risk of developing SBE
2. Burns
3. Operations involving contamination e.g., colon surgery
4. Following trauma with contaminated wounds
5. Operations involving insertion of artificial materials e.g., hip replacement, arterial grafts

Conditions predisposing to gas gangrene
1. Extensive devitalisation of muscle mass especially buttock, thigh, shoulder
2. Impaired arterial supply e.g., arterial injury/compression/peripheral vascular disease
3. Contamination by soil, clothing
4. Criminal abortion
5. Puerperal infection
6. Diabetic foot
7. Gross contamination during bowel surgery

Dermatology

EXAMINATION OF A LUMP
1. Position, shape, size, colour
2. Consistency, attachments, edge, surface
3. Tenderness, temperature
4. Pulsatility, bruit
5. Cough impulse
6. Transillumination
7. Regional lymph nodes

Lipoma. Most common lump

SEBACEOUS/EPIDERMOID CYSTS
1. Site e.g., scalp, face, scrotum, vulva, ear, back especially
2. Physical examination e.g., fluctuant, attached to skin, may have punctum
3. Complications e.g., infection, ulceration, calcification, horn formation, malignant change very rare
4. Treatment e.g., excision, including entire capsule

COMMON SITES FOR GANGLIA
1. Wrist
2. Dorsum of foot
3. Flexor aspect of fingers
4. Peroneal tendons

PILONIDAL SINUS
Most commonly found in natal cleft, but may occur:
1. Axilla
2. Umbilicus
3. Amputation stump
4. Between fingers
5. On genitalia

NAIL BED LESIONS
1. Haematoma
2. Exostosis
3. Malignant melanoma
4. Glomus tumour

FACTORS PREDISPOSING TO SQUAMOUS CELL CARCINOMA
1. Senile keratosis
2. Bowen's disease
3. Lupus vulgaris
4. Sun, X-rays
5. Pitch, tar, soot, smoking
6. Marjolin's ulcer

BASAL CELL CARCINOMA
1. 90% on face
2. Rolled pearly edge appearance
3. Central ulceration with scabbing

Treatment:
Local excision, or irradiation

MARJOLIN'S ULCER
Malignant change in ulcer, scar, sinus
1. Slow growing
2. Painless
3. Slow lymphatic spread

DIFFERENTIAL DIAGNOSIS OF MALIGNANT MELANOMA
1. From benign naevae: intradermal—compound—juvenile—junctional
2. Seborrheic keratosis
3. Sclerosing angioma
4. Pyogenic granuloma
5. Pigmented basal cell carcinoma

Which pigmented lesions should be removed?
1. Any mole undergoing change
2. Naevae in areas subjected to trauma
3. Black moles greater than 0.5 cm in diameter especially leg/back
4. Naevae on soles of feet, mucous membranes, genitalia
5. Moles on anxious patients with bad family history
6. Children with solitary growing mole
7. Those causing cosmetic problems

Signs of malignant change
1. Increase in size
2. Increase in pigment
3. Areas of depigmentation
4. Ulceration or bleeding
5. Irritation
6. Satellite lesions and spread of pigment from edge of lesion
7. Regional lymph node enlargement—distant metastases

Surgical management of melanoma
1. In absence of distant metastases the primary melanoma should be excised widely (5 cm margin all round) down to the deep fascia. A split thickness skin graft taken from the opposite side (to avoid implanting intradermal metastases) is applied to defect. Optimal excision margin is controversial
2. Management of regional lymph nodes is controversial
   (i) Elective regional lymph node excision is removal of clinically uninvolved nodes draining area of primary
   (ii) Therapeutic regional lymph node excision is removal of clinically involved nodes—this is generally recommended in absence of other spread

Indications for considering elective regional lymph node dissection
1. Primary in immediate vicinity of lymph node (neck)
2. Large ulcerating/rapidly growing lesion
3. Deep dermal or lymphatic involvement from histology of primary

Contraindications to elective regional lymph node dissection
1. A primary with an unpredictable lymph node drainage e.g., back
2. A primary far removed from regional lymph node e.g., lower leg
3. Slow growing, flat, non ulcerated primary
4. Microscopically superficial lesion (Clark I/II)
5. Patient in poor general health

Immunotherapy
Role of BCG in therapy not yet proven

Chemotherapy
For disseminated disease

Excision of solitary metastases
In lung and brain has been done rarely

Prognostic factors
level of invasion is most important

Poor prognostic factors
1. Males
2. Elderly
3. Fast growth rate
4. Pedunculated lesions
5. Lesion 2 cms/larger
6. Regional lymph node involvement
7. Lesions on the face and trunk
Metastases may appear after a delay of many years

Head and neck

DIFFERENTIAL DIAGNOSIS OF TONGUE ULCER
1. Traumatic
2. Aphthous
3. Carcinoma
4. Syphilitic
5. Tuberculous

DIFFERENTIAL DIAGNOSIS OF COMMON LIP LESIONS
1. Traumatic
2. Molluscum sebaceum
3. Papilloma
4. Herpes simplex
5. Carcinoma
6. Syphilitic

RISK FACTORS IN OROPHARYNGEAL CANCER
1. Sunlight (lip)
2. Smoking
3. Leukoplakia
4. Alcoholism
5. Chewing of tobacco or Betel nuts
6. Chronic sepsis
7. Iron deficiency—post cricoid carcinoma
8. Syphilis

Treatment of oropharyngeal squamous cell carcinoma
(Great majority)
1. Primary lesion—irradiation—external beam, interstitial; or preoperative irradiation and resection
2. Regional lymph nodes—radical neck dissection if nodes clinically involved and no evidence of further spread

FEATURES OF CARCINOMA IN PARTICULAR SITES

1. Lip
- (i)   93% affects lower lip
- (ii)   5% affects upper lip
- (iii) 2% affects angle of mouth—worse prognosis

2. Tongue
- (i)   Tip/free border most frequently involved
- (ii)   Palpation often reveals ulcer is 'tip of an iceberg' i.e., extensive deep involvement
- (iii) 40% have involved lymph nodes—especially posterior $\frac{1}{3}$ lesions

Submental—from tip
Submandibular—from sides

Treatment may involve partial mandibulectomy if periosteal lymphatics are involved. Lesions of the posterior third of the tongue have worse prognosis. May present with pain referred to ear

3. Tonsil
- (i)   Often causes persistent 'sore throat'
- (ii)   85%—squamous cell carcinoma
- (iii) 15%—lymphosarcoma

4. Nasopharynx
Differential diagnosis of lesions
- (i)   Hypertrophied lymphatic tissue (adenoids), or lymphoma
- (ii)   Juvenile angiofibroma
- (iii) Rathke's pouch cyst—craniopharyngioma
- (iv)   Dermoids
- (v)   Mixed tumours
- (vi)   Carcinoma

Symptoms of nasopharyngeal lesions.
- (i)   Nasal stuffiness,
- (ii)   Deafness (blocked eustachian tubes),
- (iii) Epistaxis (especially angiofibroma),
- (iv)   Dysphagia,
- (v)   Facial pain

Spread of malignant disease can cause III, IV, V, VI–cranial nerve palsies
Presents late—difficult area to examine

5. *Maxillary sinus*
May present with
    (i)   Nasal discharge (bloody/purulent)
    (ii)   Epiphora
    (iii) Facial swelling
    (iv) Proptosis
    (v)   Diplopia
    (vi) Palatal ulceration

6. *Larynx*
Exclude in every case of hoarseness
Differential diagnosis
    (i)   Polyp
    (ii)   Vocal nodule
    (iii) Retention cyst
    (iv) Leukoplakia
    (v)   Papillomas
Treatment
    (i)   Carcinoma—limited to true cord—deep X-ray therapy
    (ii)   Carcinoma—extending beyond true cord   ⎤ Laryngectom
            —recurrent following X-ray therapy ⎟ followed by
                                              ⎦ radiotherapy
    (iii) Neck dissection in those cases with involved nodes

CAUSES OF PAROTID SWELLING
  1. Tumours
    (i)   Mixed tumours
    (ii)   Adenolymphoma
    (iii) Carcinoma
  2. Parotitis
    (i)   Mumps
    (ii)   Postoperative and debilitated patients.
    (iii) Chronic recurrent
    (iv) Calculi.
  3. Mikulicz' syndrome
    (i)   Sarcoid
    (ii)   Reticulosis
    (iii) Sjogren's syndrome
    (iv) TB

Examination of parotid gland must include
    (i)   Palpation of gland
    (ii)   Test VII nerve
    (iii) Palpate regional lymph nodes
    (iv) Visualise and compress duct orifice
    (v)   Palpate fauces for deep involvement

Differential diagnosis of parotid swelling
   (i)   Parotid lesion
   (ii)   Sebaceous cyst
   (iii) Lipoma
   (iv) Lymph node
   (v)   Adamantinoma
   (vi) Neuroma (VII)

Features suggesting carcinoma
   (i)   Pain
   (ii)   Rapid growth
   (iii) Lymphadenopathy
   (iv) VII nerve palsy

Features of mixed tumours
   (i)   90% occur in parotid—most in superficial portion
   (ii)   If enucleated will recur
   (iii) Can undergo malignant change
   (iv) Tend to present under 50 years of age

Features of adenolymphoma
   1. Present after 50 years of age, usually
   2. 10% are bilateral
   3. May feel cystic

Treatment of parotid tumours
   1. Mixed tumour and adenolymphoma
      (i)   Superficial parotidectomy with sparing of facial nerve
   2. Carcinoma
      (i)   Parotidectomy with sacrifice of VII nerve and nerve graft
      (ii)   Irradiation
      (iii) Neck dissection if clinically involved nodes

STRUCTURES MISDIAGNOSED AS LYMPH NODES
   1. Carotid bulb
   2. Tip of Hyoid bone
   3. Posterior belly of omohyoid
   4. Transverse process C_2
   5. Cervical rib

Thyroid

PHYSICAL EXAMINATION OF PATIENT WITH THYROID DISEASE
1. *General inspection*
   (i) Does patient appear hyper/hypo/euthyroid?
   (ii) Note voice, skin, hair, eyes, hoarseness, stridor

2. *Palpation*
   (i) Pulse: tachycardia, atrial fibrillation, tachycardia during sleep
   (ii) Trachea: deviation?
   (iii) Goitre: smooth? nodular? moves on swallowing?
   (iv) Cervical lymph nodes

3. *Auscultation*
   Bruit of Grave's disease

4. *Indirect laryngoscopy*
   To exclude recurrent nerve involvement

SOLITARY THYROID NODULE
1. 25% of truly solitary nodules are malignant
2. 50% of patients with solitary nodule by clinical examination are found at surgery to have other nodules

In the elderly hypo and hyperthyroidism may have atypical presentations. Therefore always consider the diagnosis

THYROID FUNCTION TESTS

1. Radioiodine uptake — normal 20–55% in 24 hours

Falsely lowered	Falsely raised
Exogenous iodine e.g., IVP	Antithyroid drugs
Administered thyroxine	Iodine deficiency

T_3 suppression of uptake is found in high normals. Failure to suppress = thyrotoxicosis

2. Scan for functional status of nodules and position of thyroid
3. Resin uptake tests influenced by variations in level of thyroid binding globulin and drugs which compéte for protein binding e.g., salicylates/epanutin

Increased TBG	Decreased TBG
Pregnancy	Nephrotic syndrome
Oestrogens	Liver disease

4. PBI or total T_4 times resin uptake = free thyroxin index—eliminates globulin variability
5. BMR, cholesterol—indirect
6. TSH assay—most sensitive index of hypothyroidism

MANAGEMENT OF HYPERTHYROIDISM
Medical
1. Children and adolescents
2. Pregnancy
3. In preparation for surgery

Results
1. 30–50% success rate at 10 years—most patients require two years of treatment
2. No means of predicting who will respond. Return of T_3 suppressibility is good index of inactivity
3. Requires close cooperation of patient
4. Drugs can cause blood dyscrasias

Radioiodine
1. Used for patients more than 45 years of age
2. Patients who relapse after surgery
3. Patients unsuitable for surgery
4. 60% incidence of hypothyroidism at 10 years and this incidence continues to increase with time

Surgery
1. Subtotal thyroidectomy carries almost no mortality and very little morbidity
2. Result is prompt
3. Relapse rate of 8% approximately
4. Hypothyroidism in 8% approximately

COMPLICATIONS OF SURGERY
At time of operation:
1. Recurrent laryngeal nerve palsy—best avoided by identifying the nerve rather than staying away from it. Bilateral damage paralyses and abductors of the vocal cords (posterior cricoarytenoids) causing airway obstruction. Unilateral damage—hoarse voice
2. Superior laryngeal nerve palsy—weak voice
3. Pneumothorax—aspiration of air into superior mediastinum
Postoperative:
1. Tetany: Damage or removal of parathyroids. Presents as perioral tingling about 36–48 hours postoperatively
2. Thyroid storm: Does not occur in patients rendered euthyroid with preoperative antithyroid drugs
3. Haemorrhage: Leads to airway obstruction and requires immediate opening of incision
Late:
1. Hypothyroidism. If operative specimen shows lymphocytic infiltration this is more likely to occur
2. Recurrence—8%

INDICATIONS FOR SURGERY OF NONTOXIC NODULAR GOITRE

1. Tracheal compression
2. Concern about possibility of carcinoma
3. Retrosternal goitre
4. Young patients—risk of haemorrhage into cyst, toxic or malignant change
5. History of irradiation to head and neck area

INDICATIONS OF CARCINOMA

1. Solitary cold nodule
2. Very hard nodule
3. Hoarseness, Horner's syndrome
4. Lymphadenopathy

Thyroid cancer is a rare disease. In young people prognosis generally good because well differentiated tumours which spread late to lymphatics predominate. Converse is true in elderly where local, lymphatic and bloodstream spread occur early and tumours tend to be anaplastic

Types of thyroid carcinoma

	Predominant age	Lymph node	Bloodstream spread
1. Papillary 60-70%	Young—less than 30	+++	+
2. Follicular 20%	Middle—more than 30	+	++
3. Medullary 3-6%	Can be familial	++	++
4. Anaplastic 10-15%	Old	++	++

Treatment
Extent of operation depends on:
1. Pathological type
2. Distribution in gland
3. Common surgical sense

Basically
1. Remove involved lobe and isthmus for unilateral low invasive disease. e.g., low grade follicular
2. Do total thyroidectomy
    (i)   For multicentre disease e.g. papillary or previous history of neck irradiation
    (ii) Familial cases of medullary carcinoma
    (iii) Invasive follicular carcinoma
    (iv) Operable anaplastic carcinoma

Role of postoperative I[131]
1. Residual tumour
2. Pulmonary metastases
3. Bone metastases
Many tumours fail to take up adequate amounts

Thyroxine. Most patients with thyroid carcinoma are placed on thyroxine to suppress any residual stimulation of tumour by TSH

DIFFERENTIAL DIAGNOSIS OF LUMP IN SIDE OF NECK
1. Sebaceous cyst
2. Lipoma
3. Lymph node
4. Thyroid/parathyroid tumour
5. Cystic hygroma
6. Carotid artery aneurysm/carotid body tumour
7. Sumandibular/parotid gland
8. Pharyngeal pouch
9. Branchial cyst

Parathyroid

DIFFERENTIAL DIAGNOSIS OF HYPERCALCAEMIA
1. Metastatic carcinomas—most common
2. Hyperparathyroidism
3. Multiple myeloma
4. Milk alkali syndrome
5. Sarcoidosis
6. Vitamin D intoxication
7. Hyperthyroidism
8. Infantile hypercalcaemia
9. Paget's disease

CAUSES OF HYPERPARATHYROIDISM
1. Primary hyperparathyroidism
   Adenoma and hyperplasia—the incidence of each is unclear.
   Adenomas 80%. Higher incidence of hyperplasia being
   reported now. Carcinoma is a rare cause. Adenomas are
   more common in lower glands.
   In familial cases multiple pathology is seen
2. Secondary hyperparathyroidism
   (i)   Chronic renal failure
   (ii) Malabsorption
3. Tertiary Hyperparathyroidism
   From long standing secondary hyperparathyroidism

Embryology
1. The lower parathyroid glands are derived along with the
   thymus from the third branchial pouch. Their final position
   can be anywhere from mandible to anterior mediastinum
2. Upper parathyroids are derived from 4th branchial pouch and
   are more constant in position

Clinical features of hyperparathyroidism
1. Renal: Stones, infection, nephrocalcinosis, polyuria
2. Bones: Pain, fractures, cysts on x-ray
3. Gastrointestinal: Peptic ulceration, constipation, pancreatitis
4. General: Lassitude, mental changes

Special tests for diagnosis of hyperparathyroidism
1. Tests used to exclude other causes of hypercalcaemia
2. PTH levels
3. Multivariate analysis, thiazide test optional
4. Steroid suppression test—will not depress calcium in primary
   hyperparathyroidism—rarely used now

Techniques for preoperative tumour localisation
None is really very good. In majority of cases do not need to be done
  1. Selective venous catheterisation and PTH assay
  2. Selective arteriograms
  3. Selenomethionine isotope scanning
  4. Pneumomediastinography

Medical treatment of hypercalcaemia
  1. Correct dehydration with normal saline
  2. Induce diuresis with saline and frusemide
  3. In patients with renal impairment phosphate infusion can be used
  4. Steroids. (Especially malignant disease)

Parathyroid surgery
Generally agreed that exposure of all 4 parathyroids should be attempted in order to decide if pathology is hyperplasia or adenoma. Frozen sections can be misleading
  1. If adenoma—remove it alone
  2. If hyperplasia—remove 3 ½ glands
Mediastinal exploration is necessary in cases when no neck pathology is found

Complications
  1. Failure to remove pathology
  2. Recurrent nerve damage
  3. Tetany
  4. Haemorrhage
  5. Hypoparathyroidism

Causes of hypercalcaemia following surgery
  1. Persistence due to failure of initial operation
  2. Recurrence
      (i)   new adenoma
      (ii) missed hyperplasia
      (iii) carcinoma
  3. Error in diagnosis

The breast

MAIN LYMPHATIC DRAINAGE OF THE BREAST
1. Laterally to axillary lymph nodes (communicate with supraclavicular)
2. Medially to internal mammary nodes

BREAST DISEASE PRESENTS WITH
1. Lump
2. Pain
3. Discharge
4. Asymptomatic screening

Differential diagnosis of lump in breast
1. Carcinoma ⎤
2. Fibroadenosis ⎬ 95%
3. Fibroadenoma ⎦

Less commonly
1. Fat necrosis
2. Cysts (chronic abscess—retention cyst)
3. Lipoma

Differential diagnosis of discharge
1. Bloodstained
   (i) Intraductal papilloma/carcinoma
   (ii) Duct ectasia
   (iii) Fibroadenosis with cysts
2. Serous
       Pregnancy
3. Brown-green
       Fibroadenosis
4. Milky
   (i) Following lactation
   (ii) Galactocoele
5. Purulent
       Abscess

Differential diagnosis of pain in breast
1. Abscess
2. Fibroadenosis
3. Carcinoma
4. Chondritis

Carcinoma of breast kills 10 000 women per year in United Kingdom

STAGING OF BREAST CANCER
Clinical—TNM Classification
- T - Primary Tumour
  - T_1 - tumour diameter 2 cm or less—not fixed. Includes Paget's
  - T_2 - tumour diameter 2-5 cm–not fixed
  - T_3 - tumour diameter more than 5 cm
  - T_4 - skin or chest wall involvement (skin tethering/nipple retraction not included
- N - Regional Lymph Node
  - N_0 - no palpable homolateral nodes
  - N_1 - mobile homolateral axillary lymph nodes
  - N_2 - fixed homolateral axillary lymph nodes
  - N_3 - homolateral supra/infraclavicular lymph nodes or oedema of arm
- M - Distant Metastases
  - M_0 - no distant metastases
  - M_1 - distant metastases

N.B. Enlarged lymph nodes may represent reactive hyperplasia. Clinical error of 20% in assessing lymph node involvement

Clinical staging supplemented by investigation: e.g., Bone scan, liver function tests

Screening for breast cancer
1. Physical examination (2 cases/1000 examinations)
2. Physical examination and mammography (13 cases/1000 examinations)

Higher risk women
1. Positive family history
2. Prior breast cancer (8%)
3. Gross cystic disease
4. Prior history of intraductal papilloma
5. Prior history of endometrial carcinoma
6. Childless women and those conceiving after the age of 30

TREATMENT OF BREAST CANCER
1. *Early Breast Cancer*
   No evidence of disease beyond $T_2 N_1$—Aim of treatment is cure
2. *Advanced Breast Cancer*
   (i)   Disease beyond $T_2 N_1$
   (ii)   Recurrent local disease
   (iii) Metastatic disease

Aim of treatment is palliation

In assessing optimal curative treatment of early breast carcinoma remember
1. Long, e.g., 20 year follow-up is necessary to assess forms of treatment and such results are not available
2. The disease kills by bloodstream spread not lymphatic spread

Generally accepted statements about treatment of early breast carcinoma
1. No other treatment has been shown to better classical radical mastectomy
2. Postoperative irradiation has not been shown to increase survival of patients who have had a classical radical mastectomy
3. Adjuvant chemotherapy seems to increase the disease free period in premenopausal women with positive nodes. Unclear effect in postmenopausal women
4. In a five year follow-up lumpectomy with axillary lymph node sampling and irradiation if nodes positive, has been shown to be as good as classical radical mastectomy
5. There is no clear advantage to supra radical mastectomy
6. Lesser procedures may eventually be shown to be as effective as radical mastectomy with long term follow-up

TREATMENT OF ADVANCED BREAST CANCER
1. *Surgical*
   (i) Excision of local disease to prevent/treat ulceration
   (ii) Relief of complications e.g., pathological fractures
2. *Irradiation*
   (i) Local recurrence
   (ii) Painful metastases
   (iii) Pathological fractures
3. *Hormonal*
   If the tumour is oestrogen receptor positive—75% of premenopausal patients respond and 60% of postmenopausal respond
   (i) Oophorectomy—pre- and early postmenopausal
   (ii) Oestrogen therapy—postmenopausal
   Try androgens if above fail
4. *Steroids*
   (i) May benefit any group
   (ii) Correct hypercalcaemia
   (iii) Decrease brain and spinal cord swelling
   (iv) Decrease bone pain
5. *Adrenalectomy or hypophysectomy*
   For patients who relapse after responding to more simple hormonal treatment
6. *Chemotherapy*
   Advanced non hormone responsive disease

Prognosis
1. 80% die in 5 years if no treatment
2. Early treatment—70% 5 year survival rate

Lymphatics and thymus

LYMPH NODES
Causes of lymph node enlargement

1. *Infections*
   (i) Local enlargement e.g., jugulodigastric node in tonsillitis
   (ii) General enlargement e.g., mononucleosis, secondary syphilis

2. *Malignancy*
   (i) Local enlargement e.g., axilla in breast cancer
   (ii) General enlargement e.g., lymphatic leukaemia, Hodgkin's

Always examine:
1. Regional nodes
2. Other nodes
3. Liver and spleen

HODGKIN'S DISEASE
Staging of Hodgkin's disease
I   Single lymph node group involved
     Single extralymphatic organ/site involved
II   Two/more lymph node groups on same side of diaphragm involved
     Localised involvement of extralymphatic organ and lymph nodes on same side of diaphragm
III Lymph nodes on both sides of diaphragm involved
IIIa No systemic symptoms
IIIb Systemic symptoms—worse prognosis e.g., fever, sweating, weight loss, itching
IV   Disseminated disease

Histological types
1. Lymphocyte dominant—favourable prognosis
2. Nodular sclerosing—favourable prognosis
3. Mixed cellularity—intermediate prognosis
4. Lymphocyte depleted—poor prognosis

Investigations used in staging
1. Blood picture, bone marrow
2. Chest X-ray: e.g., Hilar nodes
3. Bone scan
4. Lymphangiogram
5. Surgery

Indications for surgery
1. Biopsy
2. Staging laparotomy
   (i)   Splenectomy
   (ii) Liver biopsy
   (iii) Node biopsy
   (iv) Tumour marking with metal clips to outline radiation portal
   (v)   Oophoropexy

Reasons for splenectomy
1. 25% of impalpable spleens have microscopic involvement i.e., increases accuracy of staging
2. Prevents radiation damage to left kidney and lung

Principles of treatment
Stages: 1.
        2.   } Radiotherapy
        3a.
        3b. } Chemotherapy
        4.

THYMUS
Myasthenia gravis—relationship to thymus
1. 15% of patients with Myasthenia Gravis have a thymoma
2. Thymectomy is especially effective in young women with a short history and no thymoma
3. 50% of thymomas are malignant and surgery has better results than radiation
4. Steroids are now being used for this disease, and thymectomy may lower steroid requirement

LYMPHOEDEMA
Causes of lymphoedema
1. Congenital
2. Following surgery e.g., lymph node dissection
3. Malignant disease e.g., arm swelling with breast cancer
4. Radiotherapy
5. Elephantiasis (filariasis)

Chest and lungs

COMPLICATIONS OF CHEST INJURIES
1. Ribs: Multiple fractures may cause flail chest
2. Pleura, lungs, bronchi: haemo/haemopneumothorax-surgical emphysema
3. Heart: Cardiac tamponade
        Cardiac rupture
        Ruptured papillary muscle
        Ruptured valve
4. Large vessels: Haemothorax
5. Oesophagus: Mediastinitis
6. Diaphragm: Herniation of viscera and injury of liver, spleen, kidneys

There may be little external evidence of chest injury despite severe internal injury. e.g., ruptured aorta. Stab wounds can penetrate diaphragm causing intra-abdominal injuries

Chest injuries—main principles of treatment
1. Airway: intubate—tracheostomy—positive pressure ventilation
2. Shock: blood
3. Chest drainage: of blood/air
4. Empty stomach: Nasogastric tube
5. Thoracotomy:
    (i)   Haemorrhage—which doesn't stop spontaneously
    (ii) Bronchial disruption
    (iii) Major vessel injury/tamponade

CAUSES OF PNEUMOTHORAX
1. Spontaneous: e.g., ruptured bulla
2. Traumatic: e.g., sucking chest wound
3. Iatrogenic: e.g., pleural tap. Lung biopsy, CVP line insertion positive pressure ventilation

Signs of tension pneumothorax
1. Increasing dyspnoea and cyanosis
2. Inequality of breath sounds
3. Increasing displacement of mediastinum
4. Increasing peripheral venous congestion
5. Decreasing chest compliance in patient's being ventilated

DIAGNOSIS OF CARDIAC TAMPONADE
1. Think of possibility
2. Rising pulse rate
3. Falling blood pressure
4. Rising JVP
5. Diminished heart sounds
6. Pulsus paradoxus
7. Increasing cardiac outline on chest X-ray
8. Ultrasound

CAUSES OF LUNG ABSCESS
1. Tumour:
   - (i) Distal to airway obstruction
   - (ii) Necrosis of tumour
2. Pneumonia:
   - (i) especially staphylococcal
   - (ii) TB
   - (iii) Actinomyocosis
3. Inhalation
   - (i) peanuts—children
   - (ii) teeth
   - (iii) vomit, pus
   - (iv) food-achalasia/pharyngeal pouch
4. Embólic
   - (i) septicaemia e.g., SBE, drug addicts
   - (ii) infected pulmonary infarction
5. Infected lung cysts
6. Penetrating trauma
7. Subphrenic abscess e.g., amoebic
8. Immunosuppression and general debility

Complications of lung abscess
1. Empyema—pyonpneumothorax
2. Cerebral abscess
3. Haemorrhage
4. Weight loss, anaemia

Treatment
1. Exclude bronchial obstruction
2. Dependent drainage, antibiotics
3. Open drainage if above fails

CAUSES OF EMPYEMA
1. Lung disease:
    (i)   Pneumonia
    (ii)   TB
    (iii) Carcinoma
    (iv)   Bronchiectasis
    (v)   Postoperative
2. Ruptured oesophagus
3. Subphrenic spread
4. Septicaema
5. Penetrating chest wound

Treatment of empyema
Acute:
1. Thoracentesis and antibiotics
2. Closed chest tube drainage if pus cannot be completely aspirated via thoracentesis
Chronic:
1. Open thoracotomy
2. Decortication later if lung fails to re-expand

TYPES OF LUNG TUMOUR
Benign:
1. Adenoma (carcinoid, cylindroma)
2. Hamartoma
3. Miscellaneous—rarer

Malignant—primary
1. Squamous
2. Undifferentiated large cell
3. Undifferentiated small cell (oat cell)
4. Adenocarcinoma
5. Alveolar bronchiolar type

Malignant—secondary
1. Breast ⎫
2. Kidney ⎪
3. Thyroid ⎬ Carcinoma
4. Testis ⎪
5. Adrenal ⎭
6. Choriocarcinoma
7. Sarcomas
8. Melanoma

EFFECTS OF BRONCHIAL CARCINOMA
1. Bronchial obstruction
   (i) collapse
   (ii) recurrent pneumonia ⎫ cough
   (iii) abscess ⎬ haemoptysis
   (iv) empyema ⎭ SOB
2. Pleural involvement
   (i) pain
   (ii) effusion
   (iii) pneumothorax
3. Neurological involvement
   (i) brachial plexus: arm pain
   (ii) sympathetic chain: Horner's
   (iii) recurrent nerve: hoarseness
   (iv) phrenic nerve: elevated diaphragm
4. Heart and pericardium:
   (i) pericardial effusion
   (ii) atrial fibrillation
5. Blood vessels: SVC obstruction
6. Oesophagus: Fistula
7. Lymphatics:
   (i) chylothorax
   (ii) lymphadenopathy
8. Blood spread:
   (i) bone: fractures
   (ii) brain: epilepsy
   (iii) liver: jaundice
9. Transcoelomic: Pleural seedlings

Associated findings in bronchial carcinoma
1. Clubbing
2. Weight loss
3. Anaemia
4. Neuropathies:
   (i) peripheral
   (ii) myelopathy
   (iii) cerebellar degeneration
   (iv) dementia
5. Myopathy
6. ACTH, PTH, ADH, secretion, etc.

Pancoast syndrome
1. Apical shadow on chest X-ray
2. Rib erosion
3. Horner's syndrome
4. Lower brachial plexus lesion

Investigation of bronchial carcinoma
1. Chest X-ray with tomograms
2. Cytology of sputum/pleural fluid
3. Brush biopsy
4. Bronchoscopy
5. Barium swallow—to show oesophageal displacement
6. Mediastinoscopy—exclude lymphatic spread

Bronchoscopy may reveal
1. Vocal cord paresis
2. Tracheal compression
3. Widening and loss of mobility of carina
4. Tumour

Treatment
1. Resectable lesions should be resected. Postoperative irradiation if mediastinal nodes positive may be beneficial
2. Irradiation for unresectable lesions and complications
   (i) Reduces haemoptysis
   (ii) Reduces bone pain
   (iii) Relieves SVC obstruction
   (iv) May relieve cough and dyspnoea

CAUSES OF PLEURAL EFFUSION
1. Serous:
   (i) Transudates:
      a. heart failure
      b. liver failure
      c. nephrotic syndrome
   (ii) Exudate:
      a. pneumonia
      b. tumour
      c. infarction (P.E.)
      d. Collagen disease
      e. subphrenic abscess
2. Purulent—see empyma
3. Haemorrhagic:
   (i) trauma
   (ii) embolus
   (iii) tumour
4. Chylous:
   (i) trauma
   (ii) tumour
   (iii) filariasis

CAUSES OF ABNORMAL MEDIASTINAL MASS ON CHEST X-RAY

1. *Superior mediastinum*
   - (i)   Thyroid
   - (ii) Aortic aneurysm
   - (iii) Parathyroid adenoma—rarely large enough

2. *Anterior mediastinum*
   - (i)   Thymoma
   - (ii) Dermoid cysts and teratomas
   - (iii) Lymphosarcoma, Hodgkin's
   - (iv) Pleuropericardial cyst

3. *Middle mediastinum*
   - (i)   Hilar lymph nodes
   - (ii) Bronchogenic cysts

4. *Posterior mediastinum*
   - (i)   Achalasia of cardia
   - (ii) Hiatus hernia
   - (iii) Neurofibroma

Vascular

CAUSES OF ARTERIAL OCCLUSION
1. Outside vessel—e.g.,
    (i)   Bone: supracondylar fracture (elbow
    (ii) Haematoma
    (iii) Plaster cast
2. In wall e.g.,
    (i)   Spasm: Raynauds, trauma
    (ii) Laceration:
          a. intimal flap
          b. transection
    (iii) Buerger's
3. In lumen e.g.,
    (i)   Thrombosis
    (ii) Embolism
    (iii) Atheroma

FEATURES OF CHRONIC IMPAIRMENT OF PERIPHERAL CIRCULATION
1. Claudication
    (i)   Hip pain: bilateral iliac occlusion
    (ii) Thigh pain: common femoral occlusion
    (iii) Calf pain: superficial femoral occlusion
2. Diminution or loss of pulses at rest or on exercise
3. Loss of hair, brittle opaque nails, muscle atrophy
4. Pallor on elevation
5. Dependent rubor
6. Slow capillary return
7. Slow healing wounds
8. Rest pain
9. Ulceration/gangrene

Management of claudication
1. Conservative treatment for vast majority. Increase in collateral flow often leads to improvement. Only 10% progress to gangrene
    (i)   Patient education—weight reduction
                            stop smoking
                            exercise programme
                            careful foot care
                            heel raise
    (ii) Control of diabetes and hypertension
2. Surgery: for very incapacitating symptoms in otherwise healthy patients

Management of patients with rest pain/gangrene
Urgent need for surgery

Operations. Based on arteriographic findings and condition of patient
1. Endarterectomy—local block
2. Profundoplasty
3. Bypass graft e.g., aorto-iliac
femoro-popliteal
axillo-femoral
femoro-femoral
4. Sympathectomy—in patients with unreconstructable situations
   (i) Increases blood flow to skin
   (ii) May diminish pain
   (iii) May limit extent of amputation required
5. Amputation:

FEATURES OF ACUTE ARTERIAL OCCLUSION
1. Pain
2. Pallor
3. Pulseless
4. Parasthesiae ⎤
            ⎬ Most significant because nerves are most
5. Paralysis ⎦ sensitive to hypoxia
6. Perishing cold

Sources of arterial emboli
1. 90% from heart
   (i) Atrial fibrillation
   (ii) Mitral valve disease
   (iii) Postmyocardial infarction
   Others
   (i) Atheromatous
   (ii) Myxoma, subacute bacterial endocarditis
   (iii) Paradoxical
Emboli tend to lodge at vessel bifurcations
70% affect lower extremity
20–25% affect brain
5–10% affect visceral arteries

Management of embolic arterial occlusion
Within 4 to 6 hours of onset of paralysis or parasthesiae muscle necrosis begins and muscles become firm to palpation. Therefore early diagnosis is essential
1. Heparinise—to prevent propogated thrombosis
2. Embolectomy—Fogarty catheter. Ensure removal of propogated thrombosis
3. Fasciotomy if muscles are oedematous
4. Continue anticoagulation

In some cases preoperative arteriogram is helpful
Embolus often reflects serious underlying disease (e.g., heart) 30% mortality rate. Acute occlusion can also be due to thrombosis in an atheromatous vessel. Treat on same principles; additional reconstructive procedure may be required

AETIOLOGY OF ANEURYSMS
1. Congenital e.g., berry aneurysms
2. Traumatic e.g., false aneurysm
3. Inflammatory e.g., subacute bacterial endocarditis
4. Degenerative e.g., atheromatous

Complications of aneurysms
1. Rupture: esp. abdominal aortic aneurysm
2. Thrombosis ⎫   —popliteal
            ⎬ esp. peripheral aneurysms—femoral
3. Embolism ⎭   —carotid
4. Infection: esp. salmonella
5. Pressure: e.g., dysphagia

Features of abdominal aortic aneurysms
1. 20% chance of rupture within 1 year of diagnosis
2. 50% chance of rupture over 5 years of diagnosis
3. Symptoms = impending rupture
   (i) Low back pain/sciatica
   (ii) Renal colic type pain
   (iii) Any acute abdominal condition

Aneurysms less than 5 cm diameter rarely rupture. Diagnosis is often delayed following failure to palpate abdomen carefully

Management
1. Elective resection if patient otherwise suitable. Less than 5% mortality
2. Emergency resection for rupture—much higher mortality

Complications
1. Renal failure
2. Declamping shock
3. Embolization
4. Colon necrosis
5. Myocardial infarction
6. Graft infection
7. Graft-enteric fistulae

Features of dissecting aneurysms
1. Hypertension with cystic medial necrosis is main predisposing factor (also Marfan's)
2. 60 to 70% originate in aorta just distal to aortic valve 25% originate in aorta just distal to left subclavian
3. Usually presents with sudden excruciating chest pain
4. Symptoms arise from complications
   (i) Rupture
      a. pericardium—tamponade
      b. mediastinum—shock
      c. peritoneum—shock
   (ii) Occlusion of vessels
      a. coronary—infarction
      b. head—stroke
      c. intercostals—paralysis
      d. renals—anuria
      e. mesenteric—infarction
      f. iliacs—ischaemic limb
   (iii) Aortic incompetence

Management
1. Hypotensive therapy if stable
2. Surgery
   (i) Aortic incompetence
   (ii) Major vessel occlusion
   (iii) Rupture

ARTERIAL INJURIES
Penetrating Trauma
1. 20% have normal pulse distal to injury
2. 30% have diminished pulse distal to injury
3. Arteriography may be useful with multiple injuries

Nonpenetrating injuries
1. Frequently from adjacent fracture fragments
2. Can cause wide area of intimal damage, with detachment, and little external sign of injury
3. Delayed diagnosis is frequent and may result in irreversible ischaemia. Therefore, high index of suspicion and repeated clinical examination required

SIGNS OF ARTERIOVENOUS FISTULA
1. Thrill
2. Dilated pulsating veins
3. Continuous murmur

Complications
1. Skin ulceration
2. Limb hypertrophy (in children)
3. Heart failure—rare
4. Subacute bacterial endocarditis—rare

TRAUMATIC RUPTURE THORACIC AORTA
1. Commonly follows decelerating type closed chest injury (e.g., motor vehicle accident)
2. Rupture occurs just distal to origin of left subclavian at site of ligamentum arteriosum
3. May be minimal clinical findings—but discrepancy between upper and lower limb pulses should suggest diagnosis
4. Chest X-ray nearly always shows abnormal contour

Management
1. Aortogram if patient is stable
2. Surgery—graft usually required

CAUSES OF SURGICALLY CORRECTABLE HYPERTENSION
1. Unilateral renal disease e.g., renal artery stenosis
2. Coarctation of aorta
3. Phaeochromocytoma
4. Conn's syndrome
5. Cushing's syndrome

CAUSES OF RAYNAUD'S PHENOMENON
(Pallor→Cyanosis→Rubor. Precipitated by cold/emotion)

Primary Raynaud's
no serious underlying disease

Secondary Raynaud's
1. Buerger's
2. Scleroderma
3. Cervical ribs
4. Vibrating tools
5. Systemic lupus erythematosis
6. Blood disorders

Management
1. Avoid cold
2. Sympathectomy for severe cases only
3. Medical: intra-arterial reserpine—controversial
4. Close follow-up since Raynaud's may precede signs of underlying disease by 3 to 5 years

ISCHAEMIC BOWEL DISEASE

Clinical features
1. Diagnosis often delayed
2. Mainly affects elderly patients
3. With/without—severe abdominal pain
4. Bloody diarrhoea
5. Shock
6. Ischaemic bowel may be visible via sigmoidoscope
7. Raised haematocrit, amylase, may be helpful

Classification
1. Acute mesenteric embolus—Atrial fibrillation
   Mural thrombus
   Atheroma
2. Acute mesenteric thrombosis—atheroma
3. Mesenteric venous thrombosis—splenectomy
   pyelophlebitis
4. Non occlusive infarction—follows sustained decrease in cardiac output e.g., hypovolaemea, myocardial infarction. Patients commonly on Digoxin
5. Ischaemic colitis: small vessel disease ranging in severity from gangrene to mild transient ischaemia with pain. Oral contraceptives implicated in some cases
6. Intestinal angina

Varicose veins

PRIMARY VARICOSE VEINS
Most common variety. Not associated with deep venous disease. Do not usually require surgical treatment

SECONDARY VARICOSE VEINS
Following deep venous thrombosis with subsequent recanalisation and valve incompetence

Complications of varicose veins
1. Much more common with secondary varicose veins
2. Haemorrhage
3. Phlebitis
4. Brawny oedema—generally implies perforator incompetence
5. Pigmentation
6. Ulceration
7. Dermatitis
   (i) Allergy to locally applied drugs
   (ii) Fungal infection
8. Cramps
9. Marjolin's ulcer (see p. 22)

Treatment of varicose veins
1. Patient education:
   Avoid prolonged standing
   Wear effective support stockings
   With secondary varicose veins it is especially important the patient understands that he has an incurable condition which if neglected will lead to stasis ulceration. Support stockings must be worn for the rest of patient's life
2. Injection therapy—for varicosities below knee
3. Sapheno-femoral disconnection and stripping, with ligation of incompetent perforators—followed by support stockings.
   Adequacy of deep veins can be assessed by patient's ability to tolerate firm support stockings rather than by Perthe's test

TREATMENT OF VARICOSE ULCER
1. If the ulcer is kept above level of the heart it will heal i.e., bed rest and elevation
2. Systemic antibiotics if infected
3. Small, clean ulcers can be managed with firm support e.g., Paste boot
4. Treatment of varicose veins and perforators followed by excision of ulcer and skin grafting may be necessary

DIFFERENTIAL DIAGNOSIS OF LEG ULCERS
1. Venous stasis ulcer
2. Ischaemic ulcer
3. Neurotropic ulcer e.g., diabetic
4. Malignant ulcer
5. Ulcers with rheumatoid arthritis, ulcerative colitis, acholuric jaundice, sickle cell disease, collagen diseases
6. Dermatitis artefacta
7. Syphilis

Oesophagus and diaphragm

CAUSES OF DYSPHAGIA
1. *Oral and pharyngeal*
   - (i) Pharyngitis N.B. Monilia post operatively
   - (ii) Retropharyngeal abscess
   - (iii) Oral carcinoma
   - (iv) Epiglottitis
   - (v) Pharyngeal pouch
   - (vi) Neuromuscular diseases

2. *Oesophageal lesions*
   - (i) Intraluminal – foreign body
   - (ii) Intramural – congenital atresia
     trauma – endoscopy
     stricture – reflux acid/bile
     malignancy
     achalasia
     Plummer Vinson syndrome
     scleroderma
   - (iii) Extraluminal – goitre (especially retrosternal)
     lymphadenopathy
     bronchial carcinoma

3. *General*
   - (i) Polio, syringomyelia
   - (ii) Myasthenia
   - (iii) Diphtheria

FEATURES OF ACHALASIA OF CARDIA
1. Failure of lower oesophagus sphincter to relax during swallowing
2. Absence of normal peristalsis in whole oesophagus
3. Degeneration of Auerbach's plexus seen in some
4. 7-fold increase in oesophageal carcinoma (Squamous cell)

Clinical presentation of achalasia
1. Intermittent dysphagia initially which becomes progressive
2. More difficulty with cold liquids initially
3. Pain is unusual except early in disease
4. Paroxysmal nocturnal coughing and aspiration occur often
5. Barium swallow shows rat tail deformity and frequently absent gastric air bubble

Treatment
1. Heller's operation – cardiomyotomy
2. Pneumatic dilatation

FEATURES OF PHARYNGEAL POUCH (ZENKER'S DIVERTICULUM)
1. Pulsion diverticulum between thyro and cricopharyngeus
2. Secondary to premature contraction of cricopharyngeus
3. Causes dysphagia, gurgling noises, aspiration and nocturnal coughing
4. Can be perforated during endoscopy

Treatment
1. Resection of diverticulum
2. Cricopharyngomyotomy

TYPES OF DIAPHRAGMATIC HERNIA
1. Hiatus hernia
   (i) Sliding – 90%
   (ii) Rolling – 10% (Paraoesophageal)
2. Anterior hernia of Morgagni
3. Posterolateral hernia of Bochdalek
4. Posttraumatic

Complications of diaphragmatic hernia
1. Hiatus hernia
   (i) Sliding—bleeding
   (ii) Rolling
      a. haemorrhage
      b. obstruction
      c. incarceration
      d. volvulus
      e. intrathoracic gastric dilatation
2. Bochdalek – cause of acute respiratory distress in newborn
3. Morgagni – sometimes symptomatic herniation of bowel, etc.
Hiatus hernia does not necessarily imply reflux. Most are asymptomatic. Many cases of reflux occur in absence of a hernia. Only 40% of patients with proven reflux (acid perfusion test/oesophagoscopy) can have this demonstrated on x-ray. In atypical cases the following tests are useful:
1. Standard acid perfusion test
2. Manometry – (distal oesophageal tone)
3. 24-hour pH monitoring of distal oesophagus

Factors thought to be important in preventing reflux
1. High pressure zone in region of cardia
   (i) No histological sphincter in.humans, but intrinsic oesophageal muscle thought to be responsive to humoral agents. e.g., gastrin
   (ii) Intra-abdominal segment of oesophagus is at positive pressure with respect to intrathoracic portion
Relative contributions of each to high pressure zone not known

2.   Other factors implicated relative importance unknown
   (i)   Acute gastroeosophageal angle forming flap valve mechanism
   (ii)   Pinchcock effect of right crus of diaphragm
   (iii)   Mucosal folds

Symptoms of reflux
1.   Heartburn
2.   Regurgitation
3.   Dysphagia
4.   Bleeding
5.   Choking
6.   Coughing

Differential diagnosis of reflux
1.   Angina pectoris
2.   Biliary disease
3.   Diverticulitis
4.   Peptic ulcer

Causes of oesophagitis
1.   Reflux
2.   Caustic/acid ingestion
3.   Infection e.g., candida, especially diabetics, steroids
4.   Prolonged vomiting
5.   Nasogastric tube
Prolonged inflammation causes stricture

Management of reflux
1.   Elevate head of bed with 6″ blocks
2.   Avoid lying/stooping after meals
3.   Avoid corsets/constricting clothing
4.   Antacids, gaviscon, maxalon
5.   Surgery (See Indications for Surgery)

Indications for surgery
1.   Ulcerative oesophagitis
2.   Bleeding
3.   Stricture
4.   Aspiration
5.   Failed medical treatment
6.   Paraoesophageal hernia – risk of complications (see earlier section)

Operation. Antireflux procedure e.g., Nissen Fundoplication. Most strictures can be progressively dilated and then antireflux procedure alone is sufficient. Severe cases require reconstruction

CAUSES OF RUPTURED OESOPHAGUS
1. Endoscopy
2. Forceful vomiting
3. Sharp ingested foreign body
4. Postoperative e.g., vagotomy, hiatus hernia repair
5. External trauma
6. Neoplasm

Clinical features
A highly lethal condition. Successful treatment depends on early diagnosis. Site of perforation and interval between perforation and diagnosis influence findings
1. Cervical perforation
    (i) cervical tenderness
    (ii) crepitation
    (iii) supraclavicular abscess – late
2. Thoracic perforation
    (i) crunching precordial sounds – mediastinal emphysema
    (ii) mediastinitis
    (iii) pleural effusion – hydropneumothorax
    (iv) empyema
3. Infradiaphragmatic – generalised peritonitis
Pain, fever, dysphagia – always present

Treatment

Cervical
1. Drainage – antibiotics
2. Some use antibiotics alone

All others
1. Close perforation (in early cases)
2. Adequate drainage
3. Antibiotics
4. Maintain nutrition

RISK FACTORS FOR OESOPHAGEAL CARCINOMA
1. Alcoholism
2. Plummer Vinson syndrome
3. Corrosive oesophagitis
4. Achalasia
5. Geographic e.g., South Africa

Pathological features of oesophageal carcinoma
1. Most occur at lower end
2. Most are squamous cell lesions – adenocarcinoma from gastric mucosa
3. Spreads up and down wall and out to lymphatics and neighbouring structures e.g., trachea

Clinical features of oesophageal carcinoma
1. Progressive dysphagia
2. Weight loss
3. Aspiration pneumonia

Diagnosis of oesophageal carcinoma
1. History
2. Endoscopy and biopsy
3. Barium swallow

Treatment of oesophageal carcinoma
Above aortic arch surgical resection is more difficult, but presently becoming increasingly successful. Most people still depending on radiotherapy for upper 1/3 lesions

Curative
Best results obtained with oesophagectomy. Continuity of gastrointestinal tract restored by oesophagogastric anastomosis or colon interposition. Adenocarcinoma is radioresistant. If nodes positive postoperative irradiation may be beneficial

Palliative
1. Radiotherapy alone
2. Insertion of tubes e.g., Mousseau Barbin/Celestin to cope with saliva – only partially successful

BARRETT OESOPHAGUS
In response to chronic reflux, squamous cell lining replaced by columnar (non-acid secreting). Ulcer can occur in abnormal lining. Stricture is common. Increased incidence of malignancy. Antireflux operation and dilatation recommended treatment

RUPTURED DIAPHRAGM
1. Follows blunt trauma usually
2. More common on left
3. Commonly part of more severe injury
4. Commonly missed and present years later with abnormal chest X-ray
5. Inspection of diaphragm should be included in exploratory laparotomy following trauma

Stomach and duodenum

FEATURES OF CONGENITAL HYPERTROPHIC PYLORIC STENOSIS
1. More common in first born male
2. Results in projectile (bile free) vomiting at 3 to 5 weeks
3. Baby is hungry, fails to thrive, constipated
4. During feeding – 90% have palpable tumour
5. Gastric peristalsis may be visible
6. Causes dehydration, hypokalaemia, hypochloraemic alkalosis
7. Managed by precise correction of fluid and electrolyte abnormalities followed by elective pyloromyotomy (Ramstedt)

PEPTIC ULCER DISEASE
Mucosal defect arising in or adjacent to acid secreting epithelium

1. *Duodenal ulcer group*
These patients as a group tend to have high normal/excess acid secretion, but there is much overlap
  (i)   Duodenal ulcers – 1st portion usually
  (ii)   Pyloric canal ulcer
  (iii) Combined gastric and duodenal ulcer
  (iv)   Stomal ulcers
  More Common
  (i)   In Gp O and nonsecretors of blood group antigens
  (ii)   With hyperparathyroidism
  (iii) Association with Zollinger-Ellison syndrome

2. *Gastric Ulcers*
  Seen generally as high lying lesser curve ulcers. These patients as a group tend to have normal or low acid secretion, but there is much overlap
  More Common
  (i)   Gp A
  (ii)   Chronic gastritis – leads to diminished mucosal resistance to acid and pepsin

Clinical features of peptic ulcer
1. Interval dyspepsia
2. Pain bears some relation to food, mostly relieved
3. Pain awakens patient at night
4. May present with complication of peptic ulcer disease and no antecedant history
5. Differentiation of anatomical site on basis of history is unreliable

Investigations
1. Barium meal – see later
2. Endoscopy – with biopsy
3. Acid secretion studies—seldom necessary
4. Gastrin assay
5. Exclude co-existing disease e.g., gallstones
6. Exclude hypercalcaemia

Management of duodenal ulcer group

1. *Long term*
   (i) Eat small amounts frequently
   (ii) Avoid stress
   (iii) Avoid ulcerogenic drugs
   (iv) Stop smoking
   (v) Cimetidine
   (vi) Elective surgery for intractible cases
   (vii) Emergency surgery for complications – see later

2. *Acute exacerbations*
   (i) Bed rest
   (ii) Antacids
   (iii) Sedation
   (iv) Cimetidine – unclear role

Elective surgery for duodenal ulcer group
Object is to reduce acid secretion with minimum morbidity and mortality, and lowest recurrent ulcer rate

1. *Vagotomy*
   (i) Abolishes neural stimulation of parietal cells. Diminishes response of parietal cells to other stimuli e.g., gastrin. Leads to gastric stasis. Troublesome diarrhoea can occur
   (ii) Trucal vagotomy must be accompanied by a drainage procedure – pyloroplasty, gastrojejunostomy
   (iii) Selective vagotomy leaves supply to liver and small bowel intact but does not seem to decrease diarrhoea. Drainage procedure required.
   (iv) Highly selective vagotomy – denervates parietal cell mass alone – pylorus innervation via anterior and posterior nerves of Latarget left intact. No drainage procedure required. Diarrhoea not a problem

2. *Antrectomy*
   Removes gastrin stimulus to parietal call

Results

Procedure	Recurrence rate 20 years
Truncal/selective vagotomy and drainage	5-25%
Highly selective vagotomy	? 5%
Vagotomy and antrectomy	1%
Partial gastrectomy	2-5%

Morbidity (e.g., weight loss, dumping) and mortality greater after gastrectomy

General conclusion
1. Patients with intractible symptoms who spontaneously request surgery generally have best result
2. Type of operation performed is best tailored to individual patient and findings at operation
   (i) Thin patients – avoid gastrectomy
   (ii) Heavily scarred duodenum – may make gastrectomy hazardous
3. Highly selective vagotomy may well be the 'ideal' operation but long term recurrence rates are not known
4. Cimetadine may decrease necessity for elective surgery

Management of gastric ulcer group
(Usually benign lesser curve gastric ulcers)

1. *Long term*
   (i) Stop smoking
   (ii) Antacids
   (iii) Carbenoxolone
   (iv) Elective surgery

Indications for surgery of gastric ulcers
1. Any question of malignancy
2. Very large ulcer – increased risk of bleeding/perforation
3. Failure to diminish in size by 50% after 3 weeks of medical treatment
4. Pyloric canal ulcer – respond poorly to medical treatment
5. Evidence of deep penetration – increased risk of bleeding/perforation
6. If associated with duodenal ulcer – tend to be recurrent
7. Recurrent ulcer

Operations for gastric ulcer
1. High lying type on lesser curve – partial gastrectomy
Results – Very low recurrence rate (<1%)
2. Low lying ulcers e.g., pyloric canal ulcer
   (i) Four quadrant biopsy of ulcer, if gastrectomy is not done
   (ii) Vagotomy and drainage/vagotomy and antrectomy/Polya

Complications of Gastrectomy
Early
1. Haemorrhage – e.g., suture line, ruptured spleen
2. Pancreatitis – 50% mortality rate
3. Duodenal stump leak
4. Afferent loop obstruction
5. Efferent loop obstruction
6. Anastomotic leak
7. Subphrenic abscess

Later
1. Dumping syndrome 5 to 10% incidence
   - (i) Early – occurs within 10 minutes of eating and lasts 40 to 60 minutes. Caused by premature entry of hypertonic fluid into jejunum
   - (ii) Late – occurs about two hours after eating – caused by hypoglycaemia secondary to excess insulin release

Clinical features of dumping syndrome
1. Weakness, sweating, pallor
2. Epigastric discomfort, borborygmi
3. Palpitations
4. Diarrhoea
2. Malabsorption
   - (i) 50% have iron deficiency anaemia
   - (ii) 30% have impaired B_{12} absorption
   - (iii) 30% have disordered calcium metabolism (osteomalacia)
   - (iv) Steatorrhoea more common after polya reconstruction secondary to
     - a. Gastric emptying and pancreatico-biliary secretions out of phase
     - b. Colonization of afferent loop by bile salt splitting organisms
3. Diarrhoea – from
   - (i) Vagotomy
   - (ii) Cathartic effect of bile salts
   - (iii) Steatorrhoea
4. Stomal ulcer – usually on jejunal side of stoma
   - (i) Causes – inadequate gastric resection/vagotomy
     long afferent loop
     antral remnant at tip of afferent loop
     Zollinger-Ellison syndrome
     hyperparathyriodism
   - (ii) Complications – haemorrhage
     perforation
     gastrojejunocolic fistula – best demonstrated by barium enema
5. Stomal obstruction e.g., by citrus fruits
6. Recrudescence of pulmonary TB
7. Increased risk of carcinoma in gastric remnant

COMPLICATIONS OF PEPTIC ULCER DISEASE
1. Haemorrhage
2. Perforation
3. Pyloric obstruction

Management
1. *Haemorrhage*
    (i)   Replacement of blood volume – CVP; Urine output
    (ii) Identification of bleeding site – endoscopy; arteriography
Most cases stop spontaneously. Mortality rate increases with age,
recurrent bleeds.
Operation: Suture ligation of artery, vagotomy and
pyloroplasty/gastrectomy

2. *Perforation*
    (i)   75% on anterior wall of 1st portion of duodenum
    (ii) Treatment – oversew perforation with patch of
          omentum. Copious peritoneal lavage. In poor risk
          patients no more should be done. In early cases, and
          cases with long antecedant history, definitive ulcer
          operation can be done. Biopsy of perforated gastric
          ulcers to exclude malignancy

3. *Pyloric obstruction*
    (i)   May be secondary to
          a. spasm – duodenitis
          b. scarring – chronic ulcer
          c. carcinoma
    (ii) Causes same electrolyte and fluid abnormalities as
          infantile form. See page 59
    (iii) Drainage operation – usually gastrojejunostomy and
          vagotomy for chronic ulcer. Duodenitis settles with
          intensive medical treatment

FEATURES OF ACUTE GASTRIC MUCOSAL EROSIONS
Superficial to muscularis mucosa

Related to
1. Stress
    (i)   Trauma
    (ii) Burns
    (iii) Operations
    (iv) Sepsis
2. Alcohol
3. Aspirin, phenylbutazone, indomethacin
Antacids may reduce incidence. Highly selective
vagotomy/cimetidine reported to have good results

GASTRIC CARCINOMA
1   20% increased risk with Gp A
2. 10% incidence with pernicious anaemia
3. 50% have achlorhydria
4. 40–70% occur in antrum

Clinical features of gastric carcinoma
1. Weight loss most common symptom
2. Pyloric outlet obstruction
3. Anorexia – especially for meat
4. Pain – late
5. Iron deficiency anaemia
6. May perforate/bleed
7. 30% have palpable mass
8. Dysphagia

Treatment of gastric carcinoma
50 to 70% have positive lymph nodes at operation – most important prognostic factor. Most people do a radical subtotal gastrectomy or palliative operations for bleeding, obstruction (oesophagus/pylorus), perforation

Signs on barium meal suggestive of carcinoma
1. Space occupying mass
2. Greater curve ulcer
3. Rigidity of adjacent gastric wall
4. Irregular/asymmetric crater
5. Mucosal folds do not radiate towards ulcer
6. Small thickened contracted stomach – Linitis Plastica
7. Fundal tumours are difficult to evaluate because of poor filling

N.B. Gastric carcinoma can fulfill radiological criteria for healing – i.e., biopsy is mandatory. It is now believed that benign ulcers never turn malignant

CAUSES OF ACUTE GASTRIC DILATATION
1. Postoperative – e.g., cholecystectomy
2. Trauma – chest/abdomen
3. Patients on positive pressure ventilators
4. Plaster of Paris jacket application

Clinical features of gastric dilatation
1. Hiccoughs
2. Periodic regurgitation
3. Hypotension, oliguria, tachycardia
4. Often delayed diagnosis

MALLORY WEISS SYNDROME
1. Massive haematemesis following forceful vomiting (Alcoholic, pregnancy, etc.)
2. Longitudinal mucosal tear at gastro-oesophageal junction

Treatment
1. Arteriographic localisation
2. Vasopressin infusion of left gastric artery
3. Most stop bleeding spontaneously
Surgery if no facilities for arteriography and bleeding continues

CAUSES OF GASTROINTESTINAL HAEMORRHAGE
1. *General bleeding disorders*

2. *Oesophagus*
   (i) Varices
   (ii) Oesophagitis
   (iii) Mallory Weiss syndrome

3. *Stomach*
   (i) Ulcer
   (ii) Erosions
   (iii) Tumours

4. *Duodenum*
   (i) Ulcer
   (ii) Ampullary tumour
   (iii) Haemobilia

5. *Small intestine*
   (i) Meckel's
   (ii) Tumour

6. *Large bowel*
   (i) Diverticulitis
   (ii) Carcinoma
   (iii) Inflammatory bowel disease
   (iv) Polyps
   (v) Haemorrhoids

7. *Aortic aneurysms and prosthetic grafts – may rupture into oesophagus or duodenum*

8. *Vascular anomalies e.g., haemangioma*

Most common causes of upper gastrointestinal bleeding
1. Peptic ulcers 80%
2. Erosions   15%
3. Varices   5%

Management
(see specific sections for different lesions)
In general:
1. Correct hypovolaemia and prevent shock – renal failure is
    main cause of mortality
2. Diagnosis: history, physical examination
3. Investigations:
    (i)   endoscopy
    (ii)   arteriography } Most successful
    (iii) barium studies
If barium studies are done initially subsequent angiogram may be
obscured by residual contrast
4. Control of bleeding
    (i)   Many stop spontaneously
    (ii)   Correct general bleeding disorders
    (iii) Selective infusion of vasopressin via catheter placed at
           arteriography
    (iv)   Operation

Bowel tumours

POLYPS

Polyp is a clinical term with no histopathological implications describing a mass of tissue arising from mucosa that protrudes into the bowel lumen

Classification	Single	Multiple
Benign	Adenomatous	Familial adenomatous polyposis coli
	Villous	Gardener's
Malignant	Adenocarcinoma	
Hamartomas	Juvenile	Peutz-Jegher
Inflammatory		Pseudopolyposis

Features of juvenile polyp
1. No malignant potential
2. Usually single and pedunculated
3. No treatment unless bleeds

VILLOUS ADENOMA
1. Presents with blood and mucus in stool
2. May cause hypokalaemia
3. 80% occur in recto sigmoid region
4. 30% actively invasive. 30% have atypical cellularity

Invasive lesions treated as carcinoma. Non-invasive lesions which are low-lying excised widely and area closely followed. Higher lesions – anterior resection

ADENOMATOUS POLYPS
1. 70% in recto sigmoid
2. Invasion of stalk by malignant cells is very rare
3. Less than 1% chance of malignancy if polyp diameter is less than 1.2 cm
4. Colonoscopic removal has facilitated management.

POLYPOID CARCINOMA

Vast majority are de novo carcinomas rather than malignant change in adenomatous polyp

HYPERPLASTIC POLYPS

Same colour as normal mucosa. Of no significance; extremely common

GARDNER'S SYNDROME
1. Autosomal dominant
2. 100% malignant potential in large bowel
3. Osteomas of mandible, skull, sinuses
4. Sebaceous cysts
5. Desmoid tumours
6. Polyps should be removed

FAMILIAL ADENOMATOUS POLYPOSIS COLI
1. Autosomal dominant
2. Polyps appear in teens
3. 100% malignant potential
4. Bleeding often heralds malignant change
5. Total colectomy or subtotal colectomy with ileo rectal anastomosis and observation of rectal stump every six months
6. Sigmoidoscopy of patient's relatives

PEUTZ JEGHER
1. Autosomal dominant
2. Polyps in large and small bowel – hamartomas
3. Melanin spots on oral mucosa
4. Malignant potential not conclusively established
5. Resection of polyps causing complications e.g., haemorrhage/obstruction

CARCINOID TUMOURS
1. Kulschitsky cell origin secreting serotonin mainly (also kallikrein, histamine)
2. Sites of occurrence: appendix 45% – 3% malignant
ileum 30% – 35% malignant
rectum 15%
Rarely bronchus, ovary, duodenum, stomach. 25% associated with another histologically distinct primary neoplasm

Features of carcinoid syndrome
(When liver metastases secrete tumour products):
1. Flushing
2. Diarrhoea
3. Asthma
4. Facial hyperaemia
5. Peripheral oedema
6. Pellagra
7. Valvular heart disease: pulmonary; tricuspid

Treatment
1. Surgical resection of as much tumour as possible
2. Methysergide

COLORECTAL CARCINOMA

Predisposing factors
1. Ulcerative colitis
2. Familial adenomatous polyposis coli
3. Gardner's syndrome
4. Adenomatous polyps
5. Villous polyps

Localization of Carcinoma
1. 70% occur in rectosigmoid area
2. 30% palpable per rectum
3. 60% visualised on sigmoidoscopy
4. 3% are multiple

Spread of carcinoma
Related to survival following surgery by Duke's classification:

A:	Tumour confined to bowel wall	80% 5 year survival rate
B:	Tumour extends across bowel wall	70% 5 year survival rate
C:	Involvement of regional lymph nodes	30% 5 year survival rate
D:	Distant metastases	less than 5% 5 year survival rate

1. Lymphatic spread to mesenteric and para aortic nodes
2. Bloodstream spread – liver and lung metastases
3. Transcoelomic spread – to ovaries – Krukenberg tumours
   – to pelvic peritoneum – palpable rectal shelf
4. Implantation at operation – reduced by no touch technique
5. Anastomotic recurrence – reduced by adequate (6 cm) margin

Carcinoma may present as
1. Rectal bleeding
2. Change in bowel habit-diarrhoea/constipation with diminished calibre of stool
3. Obstruction – especially left-sided lesions
4. Perforation – free or with abscess formation
5. Nagging pain, anaemia, weight loss – especially right-sided lesions
6. Fistulisation to stomach/bladder
7. General cachexia, ascites, jaundice

Investigation for colon cancer
1. Occult blood
2. Sigmoidoscopy/colonoscopy
3. Barium enema
4. IVP

Treatment

Unobstructed case
1. Mechanical bowel preparation
2. Prophylactic antibiotics (reduce incidence of wound infection)
3. Exploratory laparotomy to determine curative/palliative surgery

Curative procedures
1. Right hemicolectomy – caecum, ascending, and hepatic flexure lesion
2. Transverse colectomy – midtransverse lesions
3. Left hemicolectomy – splenic flexure, descending lesions
4. Sigmoid colectomy – sigmoid lesions
5. Anterior resection – rectosigmoid lesions
6. Abdominoperineal resection – low rectal lesions

Palliative procedures
1. Local excision of tumour to prevent further bleeding and development of obstruction
2. Cautery of low rectal tumours to avoid abdominoperineal resection and colostomy in elderly

Obstructed cases
Initially decompressed with caecostomy or transverse colostomy
Resection at later date if possible

Recurrent cases
Sometimes a treatable lesion is present e.g., new primary

Chemotherapy
Use controversial

X-Ray therapy
Use controversial. Preoperative irradiation for rectal carcinoma being used more frequently

Inflammatory bowel disease

CROHN'S DISEASE

Transmural granulomatous inflammatory disease. Thickened bowel.
Mesenteric fat covering serosa. Enlarged mesenteric nodes,
adhesions and fistulae. Mainly submucosal thickening with mucosal
nodularity and ulcers. Skip lesions common. May have infective
aetiology. Increasing incidence

    50% terminal ileal involvement only
    30% have large and small bowel involvement

Peak onset 27 years. Large bowel involvement more common in
elderly. Can be difficult to differentiate from ulcerative colitis

Complications

Local
    Obstruction
    Perforation with abscess
    Perianal abscess/fistula
    Fistulae – bowel, bladder, vagina

General
    Malabsorption: Iron, B_{12}, vitamin D, fats
    Polyarthritis, ankylosing spondylitis
    Erythema nodosum, pyoderma gangrenosum
    Fatty liver, pericholangitis, portal fibrosis, gallstones
    Uveitis
    Periureteric fibrosis, right hydronephrosis
    Carcinoma of small and large bowel (20 fold increase)
    Amyloidosis

Common presenting features
1. Majority – insidious onset pain
2. Partial small bowel obstruction
3. Diarrhoea in 85%
4. Fever in 30%
5. Fistulae – vaginal/vesical
6. 10% with acute onset disease mimicking appendicitis with palpable mass in right lower quadrant

Diagnosis
1. Barium visualisation of small and large bowel showing narrowing (Kantor's string sign), fistulae, e.g., skip lesions
2. Biopsy per sigmoidoscope/gross appearance of mucosa
3. B_{12} absorption studies
4. At laparotomy

Management
Very sound doctor-patient relationship
Symptomatic:
    Pain – avoid addicting drugs
    Diarrhoea
    Malabsorption—Iron, B_{12}
Specific:
1. Salazopyrin
2. Steroids
3. Azothaprin – ineffective

Indications for Surgery
Obstruction – (after trial of steroids)
Abscess
Fistulae – depending on clinical features and site e.g., vesico-colic.
                Treat patient not X-ray appearance
Severe perianal disease
Severe systemic complications
Failure of medical treatment

Operation
Small bowel: Resection
Large bowel: Panproctocolectomy with ileostomy has lowest recurrence rate, but more conservative operations are done for localised disease
About 70% of cases eventually require surgery

ULCERATIVE COLITIS
Clinical features of ulcerative colitis
May be fulminant, chronic, relapsing. Tenesmus, profuse diarrhoea with blood, pus, mucus. Dehydration, systemic toxicity, depending on form

Pathological features
Primarily affects mucosa and submucosa with inflammatory cell infiltrate, crypt abscess, and ulcer formation
Redundant mucosa between ulcers forms pseudopolyps. Results in hyperaemic friable mucosa with contact bleeding
No skip areas. Rectosigmoid area most commonly involved – in half cases total colonic involvement. Chronic disease causes shortening and thickening of bowel wall with haustral loss
Disease tends to 'burn out' leaving thinned atrophic bowel

Complications of ulcerative colitis

Local
Perforation –
Megacolon
Stricture
Carcinoma

General
Weight loss, anaemia, electrolyte disorders, hypoproteinaemia
Arthritis ankylosing spondylitis
Iritis
Fatty liver, hepatitis, cirrhosis
Pyoderma gangrenosum, erythema nodosum

Features of toxic megacolon
2–5% incidence
1. Usually occurs with initial acute episode
2. May be precipitated by barium enema, anticholinergics, morphine
3. Suspect if patient with acute colitis has a sharp decrease in number of stools without improvement in general condition
4. Abdominal distension may be only physical sign
5. X-ray shows dilated colon. 10 cm or greater on X-ray is considered critical
6. If untreated will rupture
7. Essentially a clinical diagnosis

Features of carcinoma complicating ulcerative colitis
1. Ten-fold increase in risk overall
2. Especially those with early onset; continued activity of disease; diffuse involvement
3. Risk increases greatly after 10 years of active disease
4. Prognosis poor (20% 5 year survival rate) because symptoms may be confused with exacerbation of colitis and carcinoma tends to be infiltrative, flat, undifferentiated, mucus secreting and multiple

Diagnosis of ulcerative colitis
1. Exclude specific causes of diarrhoea e.g., bacillary, amoebic
2. Sigmoidoscopy and biopsy
3. Differentiation from Crohn's disease

Management
85% cases medical
1. Antidiarrhoel agents, codeine, lomotil
2. Salazopypin
3. Steroids
    (i)   Improve clinical state
    (ii) Can mask perforation
    (iii) Morbidity of surgery increased
    (iv) Patients should be weaned off steroids as soon as possible
    (v)   Steroid enemas of use with left-sided colitis
4. General nutrition, iron, vitamins
5. Regular sigmoidoscopy and barium enemas to detect malignancy

COMPLICATIONS OF STOMAS (ILEOSTOMY AND COLOSTOMY)
Most arise from incorrect placement on abdominal wall and poor technique
This is the most important part of the operation for the patient. He lives with his stoma
Preoperative selection of stoma site with patient's cooperation is essential
Must avoid having stoma close to bony prominences, or in skin fold (absent in supine position)

Specific Complications
1. Retraction
2. Stenosis
3. Skin excoriation
4. Parastomal hernia
5. Lateral space obstruction (Internal hernia)
6. Perforation

Diverticular disease

Aetiology
It is postulated that a low residue diet leads to hypersegmentation and hypertrophy of circular muscle. Increased intraluminal pressure forms pulsion diverticula. Dietary bran lowers intraluminal pressure, and may reduce tendency to diverticulum formation

Complications of diverticular disease
1. Diverticulitis – left-sided 'appendicitis'
2. Haemorrhage – more than 50% from ascending and proximal transverse colon
3. Fistulae into bowel, bladder, uterus, vagina, etc.
4. Stricture
5. Small bowel obstruction – secondary to adhesions
6. Misdiagnosis of carcinoma

X-Ray features of diverticular disease
1. Usually involves long segment
2. Funnel-shaped transition from normal to diseased bowel
3. Spasticity relieved by i.v. glucagon
4. Saw tooth pattern of mucosa may be seen
5. Intramural fistulae – evidence of diverticulitis
Carcinoma usually involves short segment of bowel and begins abruptly.
Differentiation may be impossible radiographically. Carcinoma and diverticular disease may co-exist

Treatment of complications
1. Acute diverticulitis: i.v. fluids and antibiotics – most cases resolve
   Increasing peritonitis (purulent/faecal) or mass (abscess) are indications for surgery

Principles of surgical treatment
    (i)   Peritoneal toilet
    (ii) Drainage
    (iii) If feasible: resection of diseased colon and creation of colostomy and mucous fistula
    (iv) **Or** transverse colostomy if resection unfeasible
2. Haemorrhage: Most stop spontaneously
   Arteriography for localisation of bleeding site
   Segmental resection if bleeding does not cease
   Subtotal colectomy if no facilities for arteriography
3. Fistula: Excision of bowel and fistula tract with closure of healthy tissues
4. Stricture: Differentiate from carcinoma and resect
5. Small Bowel Obstruction: Lyse adhesions

Perianal disease

CONDITIONS CAUSING ACUTE PERIANAL PAIN
1. Thrombosed haemorrhoids
2. Perianal haematoma
3. Fissure – in – ano
4. Perianal/rectal abscess
5. Proctagia fugax (actually rectal pain)

The management of a patient with perianal pain must always take into consideration possible underlying diseases such as Crohn's, ulcerative colitis, carcinoma

Complications of haemorrhoids
1. Bleeding
2. Mucous discharge and pruritis ani
3. Thrombosis
4. Ulceration

Management of haemorrhoids
1. Bran in diet, suppositories
2. Rubber band ligation
3. Injection
4. Anal stretch
5. Haemorroidectomy – severe cases only

Anal fissure
Features seen as triad:
(i)   sentinal skin tag
(ii) hypertrophied anal papilla
(iii) anal ulcer

Mostly occur posteriorly in midline – any position off midline especially oedematous and indolent fissures may represent Crohn's/ulcerative colitis
In unusual fissures also consider:
(i)   epidermal carcinoma
(ii) TB
(iii) syphilis

Management of fissure
1. Trial of stool softener
2. Anal stretch
3. Partial spincterotomy

ANO-RECTAL ABSCESS AND FISTULA

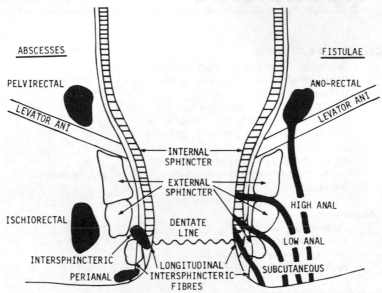

Initial step in pathogenesis is formation of abscess in anal gland between internal sphincter and longitudinal intersphincteric muscle fibres. Pus tracks up/down to locations in diagram. A fistula is an inflammatory tract with external opening in skin and internal opening in mucosa of anus/rectum. Fistula originates in an abscess

Management

Abscesses
Incision and drainage even if no fluctuance – localised tenderness on examination is sufficient. In perianal abscesses a probe may reveal internal opening which can also be laid open

Fistulae
May follow drainage of abscess. Should be laid open, avoiding damage to ano-rectal ring. Can be very complex

Causes of pruritis ani
1. Poor anal hygiene
2. Redundant mucosa, fissures
3. Contact dermatitis, eczema
4. Diabetes, Hodgkin's
5. Monilia, worms, pediculosis

Appendicitis

CLINICAL FEATURES
1. Anorexia: usually first sign – not invariable
2. Pain: Initially central (visceral) then migrates to site of inflamed appendix (parietal)
   Retrocaecal: flank/back pain
   Pelvic: suprapubic pain – dysuria
   Postileal: testicular pain – diarrhoea
3. Vomiting
4. Fever: low grade unless perforation
5. Leukocytosis: variable – should not influence diagnosis or management

Complications
1. Perforation with
   (i) Abscess formation
   (ii) Generalised peritonitis
2. Pyelophlebitis and liver abscess – rare

Differential diagnosis
From any acute abdominal condition. In very young and very old presentation may be atypical with misleading abdominal signs. Delay in diagnosis increases incidence of perforation which in turn increases mortality 30 times. Diagnosis is a clinical one and it is better to remove a normal appendix than allow perforation to occur. Importance of rectal examination in detection of pelvic tenderness cannot be overemphasised

Specific differentiation from
1. Acute mesenteric adenitis
2. Gastroenteritis
3. Urinary tract infection
4. Pelvic inflammatory disease
5. Ovarian cyst complication (torsion, haemorrhage, rupture, incarceration)
6. Ruptured ectopic pregnancy
7. Perforated peptic ulcer
8. Perforated caecal carcinoma
9. Cholecystitis, diverticulitis
10. Testicular torsion
11. Crohn's disease
12. Meckel's diverticulum
13. Henoch Shonlein purpura
14. Basal pneumonia/pleurisy
15. Zoster
16. Trauma: history may be forgotten especially by children

Management
1. Preoperative resuscitation of sick patients to correct hypovolaemia, electrolyte disorders, diabetes
2. Acute appendicitis without rupture: appendicectomy
3. Acute appendicitis ruptured with generalised peritonitis – appendicectomy, peritoneal toilet, antibiotics, drainage (optional)
4. Appendix phlegmon – i.e., non fluctuant mass – do not disturb – close – do interval appendicectomy – examination under anaesthesia can reveal mass prior to incision
5. Appendix abscess – drain – interval appendicectomy
6. Appendix mass evident on initial clinical examination in nontoxic patient – i.v. fluids – monitor size of mass. Most resolve. If systemic toxicity develops or mass enlarges – drain – interval appendicectomy. Do barium enema to exclude colon neoplasm/Crohn's

Causes of a mass in right lower quadrant
1. Appendix
2. Caecal carcinoma
3. Crohn's, TB, actinomycosis, amoebiasis
4. Psoas abscess
5. Pelvic kidney
6. Ovarian cyst
7. Lymphoma
8. Aneurysm (iliac artery)
9. Foreign body perforation

Peritonitis

CAUSES OF PERITONITIS
Intra-abdominal viscus
   Appendicitis
   Perforated peptic ulcer
   Cholecystitis
   Diverticulitis
   Ischaemic bowel
   Anastomotic leak
   Pancreatitis
Ascending
   Acute salpingitis
   Post partum infection
External source
   Penetrating trauma
   Postoperative
   Starch
Haematogenous spread
   Pneumococcal
   Streptococcal
   Staphylococcal
   TB

Course of peritonitis
   1. May be walled off by omentum and adjacent viscera and resolution may occur
   2. May be walled off and lead to abscess formation
   3. May become generalised

Pathological features of generalised peritonitis
   1. Systemic toxicity – in the elderly and patients on steroids, usual fever, leukocytosis, may be absent
   2. Sequestation of fluid within distended adynamic bowel and in peritoneal exudate
   3. Respiratory failure from diaphragm elevation and fixation, and septicaemia, leading to acidosis and hypoxaemia
   4. Renal failure – largely prerenal from dehydration. Increasing acidosis

Clinical features of peritonitis
1. Sharp pain – worse on movement/coughing
2. Pain may be referred to shoulder – diaphragmatic irritations
3. Vomiting and distension
4. Guarding and percussion/or rebound tenderness
5. Bowel sounds diminished – unreliable
6. Pelvic peritonitis may manifest as diarrhoea dysuria/frequency. Rectal examination essential to elicit tenderness of pelvic peritoneum
7. In elderly and those on steroids signs may be very subtle. Therefore, high index of suspicion is essential

Diagnosis of peritonitis
1. Essentially a clinical diagnosis
2. Upright/lateral decubitus x-rays may reveal free air indicative of perforation. Patient should be in position for 10 minutes prior to film
3. Peritoneal lavage may be useful in difficult cases

Management
1. Diagnosis
2. Volume replacement – best monitored by CVP, haematocrit, urine output
3. Nasogastric suction
4. Antibiotic therapy: some emphasis now being placed on giving adequate anaerobic cover in situations where anaerobic infection is likely e.g., perforated appendix, diverticulum. e.g., with chloramphenicol/clindamycin/metronidazole. Broad gram – ve coverage essential e.g., kanamycin, gentamycin. Antibiotics and adequate drainage at operation, are complementary
5. Surgery: depending on diagnosis. e.g. closure of perforation, appendicectomy. Sump drainage better than simple drain

Primary pneumococcal/streptococcal peritonitis
1. Usually seen in children
2. Patients with nephrotic syndrome at greater risk
3. More common with cirrhosis and ascites
4. Peritoneal tap and gram stain may enable diagnosis
5. Increased incidence following splenectomy

Features of TB peritonitis
1. Associated with focus in lungs, gut, mesenteric nodes.
2. Dry form seen as adhesions with tubercles
3. Wet form seen as ascites
4. On palpation abdomen is said to be 'doughy'

Starch peritonitis
1. Follows surgery 10 days to 3 weeks
2. Low grade fever
3. Pulse frequently out of proportion to fever
4. Mass may be palpable
5. Granulomas seen on microscopy
6. Peritoneal tap reveals – birefringent granules
7. Steroids, indomethacin useful

Sites for intra abdominal abscess
1. Right and left subphrenic spaces
2. Subhepatic space
3. Lesser sac
4. Pouch of Douglas
5. Right and left paracolic gutters
6. Around diseased viscera e.g.,
    (i)   periappendiceal
    (ii) pericholecystic
    (iii) pericolic
    (iv) tubo-ovarian
    (v)   interloop

Clinical features of intra-abdominal abscesses
1. General malaise, fever, weight loss. Failure to progress following surgery
2. May have hiccoughs/shoulder pain
3. May have palpable mass per abdomen/rectum
4. Remember pus somewhere, pus nowhere, pus under the diaphragm

Investigations in subphrenic abscess
1. Elevation and fixation of diaphragm on affected side shown by fluoroscopy
2. Sympathetic pleural effusion
3. Gas/fluid level below diaphragm
4. Simultaneous lung/liver scan for abnormal separation
5. Gallium scan being used with some success in identifying collections of pus anywhere

Management of intra-abdominal abscess
Mainstay of treatment is adequate drainage. Antibiotics may be used in addition

Intestinal obstruction

CAUSES OF INTESTINAL OBSTRUCTION
1. *Intraluminal*
    (i)   Meconium
    (ii) Intussusception
    (iii) Gallstones
    (iv) Impactions, faecal, worms, barium, bezoar, food e.g., citrus in gastroenterostomy

2. *Bowel Wall*
    (i)   Congenital:
          a. atresia, stenosis
          b. imperforate anus
          c. duplications
          d. Meckel's
    (ii) Traumatic:
          a. Haematoma
          b. Stricture
    (iii) Inflammatory:
          a. Crohn's
          b. diverticulitis
    (iv) Neoplastic
    (v)   Miscellaneous:
          a. K+ induced stricture
          b. radiation stricture
          c. endometriosis

3. *Extraluminal*
    (i)   Adhesions/bands
    (ii)   Hernia
    (iii) Annular pancreas
    (iv)   Anomalous vessels
    (v)   Absnesses
    (vi)   Haematoma
    (vii) Neoplasms
    (viii) Volvulus

Adhesions ⎫
Hernias   ⎬ Account for 80% of cases
Carcinoma ⎭

Types of obstruction
1. Simple
2. Strangulated
3. Closed loop
4. Partial/complete
5. Large bowel
6. Small bowel

Clinical features
1. Pain – usually crampy
2. Vomiting
3. Constipation – faeces/flatus
4. Distension

Management
1. Decompression – nasogastric tube – long tube
2. Volume and electrolyte replacement
3. Surgery

Surgical procedures
1. Lysis of adhesions
2. Reduction/resection of intussusception
3. Reduction hernia
4. Enterotomy – removal of gallstone/bezoar
5. Resection of obstructing lesion/strangulated bowel
6. Bypass
7. Untwisting of volvulus
8. Decompression with proximal ostomy:
   (i)   ileostomy
   (ii) caecostomy
   (iii) colostomy

Indications for emergency surgery
1. Strangulation
2. Closed loop
3. Colon obstruction
4. Early simple mechanical obstruction, unless cause, e.g., Crohn's is known

There is no reliable clinical means of excluding the presence of strangulated bowel. Management depends on striking a balance between adequate preoperative resuscitation, and operating in time to prevent strangulation or perforation. The longer obstruction has been present, the longer the resuscitation period required to avoid intraoperative hypotension and renal failure

AETIOLOGY OF PARALYTIC ILEUS
1. Postoperative
2. Peritonitis
3. Retroperitoneal haemorrhage, fractured vertebrae
4. Ureteric colic
5. Hypokalaemia
6. Hypomagnasaemia
7. Uraemia
8. Diabetic coma
9. Drugs e.g., probanthine
10. Hypothyroidism
11. Spinal cord injury

Clinical features of paralytic ileus
1. Little/no abdominal pain
2. Abdominal distension
3. Failure to pass flatus/faeces
4. No local abdominal tenderness
5. Vomiting/persistent high nasogastric drainage
6. X-rays show gas throughout small and large bowel (does not exclude partial mechanical obstruction)

Management
1. Depends on cause
2. Nasogastric suction
3. Correction of fluid/electrolyte disorder
4. Surgery if correctable cause

FEATURES OF INTUSSUSCEPTION
1. 95% occur in children – no underlying cause
2. In adults – polyp, carcinoma or Meckel's is generally initiating factor
3. Children scream and become pale with colic
4. Red currant jelly stool
5. Sausage-shaped tumour palpable in 90% of cases per abdomen/rectum

Management
1. Attempted barium enema reduction in children
2. Surgery in adults – usually resection because high incidence of associated pathology

MECKEL'S DIVERTICULUM
1. May contain ectopic gastric/pancreatic tissue
2. Present in 2% population 2 ft above ileocaecal valve
3. Can sometimes be shown using tecnetium scan

Complications
1. Diverticulitis
2. Bleeding
3. Obstruction
   (i) intussusception
   (ii) volvulus

Liver

CAUSES OF HEPATOMEGALY:

1. *Neoplastic*
   - (i)   Metastases
   - (ii) Hepatoma
   - (iii) Lymphoma

2. *Inflammatory*
   - (i)   Hepatitis
   - (ii) Hepatic abscess
   - (iii) (Leptospirosis, Actinomycosis)

3. *Parasitic*
   - (i)   Amoebic hepatitis
   - (ii) Hydatid

4. *Cirrhosis*
   see later

5. *Venous congestion*
   - (i)   Congestive cardiac failure
   - (ii) Hepatic vein thrombosis

6. *Haemopoetic*
   - (i)   Leukaemia
   - (ii) Polycythaemia
   - (iii) Myelofibrosis

7. *Metabolic*
   - (i)   Amyloid
   - (ii) Storage diseases

8. *Congenital*
   - (i)   Riedel's lobe
   - (ii) Polycystic

CLASSIFICATION OF JAUNDICE

1. *Prehepatic*
   Haemolysis
   - (i)   hereditary spherocytosis
   - (ii) G6PD deficiency
   - (iii) blood transfusions

2. *Hepatic*
   Hepatitis
   Cirrhosis
   Drugs
   Liver tumour

3. *Posthepatic* – (Obstructive)
   Stone
   Stricture
   Tumour
   (i)   pancreas
   (ii) bile duct
   (iii) nodes
   Pancreatitis

In practice intra and extra hepatic cholestasis can be difficult to differentiate. See note on ERCP and percutaneous transhepatic cholangiogram (Page 93)

Causes of pyogenic liver abscess
1. Ascending biliary infection
2. Haematogenous infection, e.g., pyelophlebitis
3. Direct extension of intraperitoneal infection
4. Trauma
5. Generalised septicaemia

Features of amoebic abscess
1. Right lobe most commonly involved
2. Associated with fever and tender liver
3. May become secondarily infected
4. May rupture into:
   (i)   pleura
   (ii) lung
   (iii) pericardium
   (iv) peritoneum
   (v)   colon
5. Treated by aspiration and metronidazole

HYDATID DISEASE OF LIVER
1. Life Cycle
   Ova in sheep offal eaten by dogs. Tapeworm develops in dog and sheds ova. Ova on contaminated vegetables, etc. eaten by man – penetrate stomach reach liver
2. Hydatid Cysts
   (i)   80% in right lobe
   (ii) calcified rim on X-ray
   (iii) Casoni test
3. Complications
   (i)   secondary infection
   (ii) rupture into pleura, biliary tree, peritoneal cavity

Rupture may be accompanied by uriticaria and other anaphylactic manifestations
Calcified cysts are inactive and no treatment required. Others should be aspirated, injected with formalin and then excised

CIRRHOSIS OF LIVER
1. Alcoholic
2. Posthepatitic
3. Idiopathic
4. Primary biliary cirrhosis
5. Secondary to chronic biliary obstruction
6. Chronic congestive heart failure – not true cirrhosis
7. Haemochromatosis
8. Wilson's disease
9. Schistosomiasis

PHYSICAL STIGMATA OF LIVER DISEASE/FAILURE
1. Jaundice
2. Spider naevae
3. White nails
4. Dupuytrens
5. Palmar erythema
6. Clubbing
7. Foetor hepaticus
8. Slurred speech
9. Flapping tremor
10. Parotid enlargement
11. Oedema
12. Gynaecomastia
13. Testicular atrophy
14. Ascites
15. Hepato-splenomegaly ⎫
                          ⎬ if with portal hypertension
    Caput medusae   ⎭

PORTAL HYPERTENSION
(more than 30 cm water)

Classification

Prehepatic
Portal vein thrombosis following:
1. Umbilical sepsis/exchange transfusion
2. Pyelophlebitis – e.g., from appendicitis/diverticulitis
3. Platelet disorder e.g., myelofibrosis/following splenectomy
4. Pancreatic tumour

Hepatic
All forms of cirrhosis

Posthepatic
1. Hepatic vein obstruction
2. Constrictive pericarditis
3. Budd Chiari syndrome
4. Veno occlusive disease

Complications of portal hypertension
1. Hypertrophy of porto systemic collaterals
   (i) Oesophageal varices
   (ii) Haemorrhoids
   (iii) Caput medusae
   and others intra abdominally which make surgery difficult
2. Splenomegaly – may lead to hypersplenism
3. Ascites
4. Hepatic failure

Clinical course of oesophageal varices
30% of patients with varices bleed. Following a bleed there is a 60% chance of a recurrence. Cirrhotics who bleed have a 70% mortality rate within a year. In patients with varices, an upper gastrointestinal bleed is due to
1. Varices in 60%
2. Gastritis in 30%
3. Duodenal ulcer in 10%
Endoscopy in expert hands after lavage through a wide bore tube is extremely accurate. Angiography can demonstrate active bleeding sites and allow superior mesenteric artery catheter placement for vasopressin infusion. Barium meal makes early angiography impossible because barium obscures the angiogram

Conservative management
1. Volume replacement:
   fresh blood (i) less ammonia
   (ii) clotting factors
2. Enemas
3. Neomycin and lactulose } to reduce Nitrogen load to liver
4. IV Vasopressin or sup. mesenteric artery infusion
5. Direct injection of bleeding varices, with sclerosing solution
6. 24 hour trial of Sengstaken tube
   Problems:
   (i) aspiration of saliva into lungs
   (ii) asphyxiation can occur if dislodgement occurs
   Pair of scissors to cut catheter and decompress balloons must be at bedside at all times for this reason
   (iii) Oesophageal and gastric pressure necrosis can occur

Surgical decompression of varices
Better prognosis if
1. Albumin more than 2.5 g/100 ml – 25Gms/1
2. Bilirubin less than 2.0 mg/100 ml – 34umol/1
3. No ascites
4. Normal prothrombin time
5. No signs of encephalopathy
No benefit shown from prophylactic shunts, largely because impossible to predict who will bleed, and 25% encephalopathy rate

Emergency surgery to stop bleeding
50% mortality
1. Graft between superior mesenteric vein and vena cava/porto-caval shunt has most acceptable mortality rate
2. Oesophageal ligation of varices has greater complication rate
3. Injection of varices has been very successful in some British centres

Elective surgery to prevent further bleeding
1. Carries lower mortality rate. Liver function can be improved preoperatively by adequate nutrition, abstinence from alcohol
2. Major emphasis is now on operations which decompress varices selectively and do not reduce hepatic flow viz Warren distal spleno renal shunt. The risk of encephalopathy is thus reduced
3. Underlying problem, however, is a poorly functioning liver, often in alcoholics, with complex social situations. Surgery may alter mode of death, but ultimately liver failure occurs

NEOPLASTIC DISEASE OF LIVER
Primary
1. Hepatoma
2. Cholangiocarcinoma
3. Adenomas – oral contraceptives

Secondary
Most common
1. From portal spread
2. Systemic: lung, breast, etc.
3. Direct: Stomach, colon, gallbladder

Aetiology of hepatoma
1. 5% incidence in cirrhotics
2. Haemochromatosis
3. Aflatoxin – dietary

Clinical features of hepatoma
1. Weight loss, malaise
2. Pain following necrosis or haemorrhage
3. Hepatomegaly
4. Ascites
5. Rapid increase in signs/symptoms of cirrhosis/haemochromatosis
6. Hypoglycaemia or improvement of diabetes
7. α Foeto protein 70% positive in Africa; 30% positive in West (Positive in any regenerative liver condition)
8. Resection is only hope of cure at present. Transplantation – experimental stages

Clinical features of secondaries in liver
1. Large hard irregular liver
2. Jaundice
3. Liver failure
4. Ascites
5. IVC obstruction with leg oedema

Secondaries are supplied mainly by hepatic artery. Ligation of hepatic artery and intra-arterial infusion of cytotoxics has been tried for treatment. 'Solitary' secondaries may be resected

Liver trauma
Often associated with injury of spleen, diaphragm, etc. Laparotomy essential.

Summary of surgical treatment

General
Correction of volume deficit
Exclusion of other injuries

Specific
1. Treatment of general bleeding diathesis
2. Direct ligature of bleeding vessels if possible
3. Ligation of hepatic artery – usually very successful
4. Lobectomy for massive damage
5. Provide adequate drainage – preferably dependent via 12th rib incision
6. Cholecystectomy may be necessary

Suturing of liver lacerations leads to fluid filled dead space. Contents may ultimately drain into biliary tree causing haemobilia or become infected. This is avoided by leaving lacerations open and providing adequate drainage. 'Over-treatment' frequently increases morbidity

Gallbladder and bile ducts

FACTORS PREDISPOSING TO GALLSTONE FORMATION
1. Lithogenic bile
2. Stasis
3. Infection
4. Haemolysis
5. Diabetes
6. Hyperlipidaemia
7. Contraceptive pill
8. Parasites – clonorchis, ascaris
9. Crohn's disease
10. Phaeochromocytoma

COMPLICATIONS OF GALLSTONES
1. Biliary colic
2. Acute cholecystitis
3. Chronic cholecystitis
4. Perforation of gall bladder and peritonitis
5. Common duct obstruction
6. Cholangitis
7. Fistulisation from biliary tree to stomach, duodenum, small bowel or colon
8. Gall stone ileus
9. Increased incidence of pancreatitis
10. Carcinoma of gall bladder

Asymptomatic stones are likely to cause complications in over 50% of patients eventually

Differential diagnosis of acute cholecystitis
1. Peptic ulcer
2. Pancreatitis
3. Appendicitis
4. Hepatitis
5. Myocardial infarction
6. Pneumonia
7. Pleurisy
8. Herpes Zoster

Clinical features of cholangitis
1. Jaundice
2. Intermittent fever ⎫ Charcot's Triad
3. Rigors ⎭

Courvoisier's law
If in the presence of jaundice the gallbladder is palpable, then a stone is not a likely cause

INVESTIGATIONS USED FOR BILIARY TRACT
1. *Plain abdominal film*
   (i) 10% of calculi are opaque
   (ii) Gas in biliary tree indicates biliary enteric fistula or infection with gas forming organisms

2. *Oral cholecystogram*
For visualisation of gallbladder which concentrates normally
Causes of nonvisualisation
   (i) Failure to absorb tablets (vomiting, diarrhoea)
   (ii) Hepatic dysfunction
   (iii) Pancreatitis
   (iv) Hepatic/cystic duct obstruction
   (v) Gallbladder dysfunction
   (vi) Elevated bilirubin

3. *Intravenous cholangiogram*
Does not depend on gall bladder concentration/absorption from gut. Visualisation of common duct without gall bladder is very good evidence for cholecystitis. Allergic reactions may occur

4. *Endoscopic retrograde cholangio pancreatography*
Gives direct visualisation of common/pancreatic duct, giving information even in jaundiced patients

5. *Ultrasound*
Can demonstrate presence of stones and size of duct system

6. *Isotope scanning:*
Being developed to help distinguish between intrahepatic and extrahepatic cholestasis (Rose Bengal)

7. *Percutaneous transhepatic cholangiography*
To distinguish intra and extra hepatic cholestasis and obtain view of duct system

Management of cholecystitis
Controversy regarding merits of early or delayed elective surgery.
Trials have shown no difference in mortality or morbidity if operation carried out within 72 hours of disease onset

Conservative management
1. Nasogastric suction
2. Intravenous fluids
3. Antibiotics
4. Analgesics (not morphine)
5. Elective cholecystectomy 2–3 months later

Indications for Early Cholecystectomy
1. Doubt about diagnosis
2. Clinical deterioration suggesting possible perforation
3. Emphysematous cholecystitis

Indications for common duct exploration
1. Jaundice
2. Palpable stones in common duct
3. Dilated common duct
4. Recurrent chills/fever suggestive of cholangitis
5. Multiple small stones in gallbladder and large cystic duct
6. Pancreatitis associated with biliary disease
7. Abnormal peroperative cholangiogram

Complications of cholecystectomy
Frequently arise from failure to recognise vascular or ductal
anomalies which are extremely common in this area
Specifically:
   (i)   Jaundice: Missed duct stone; ligature of common duct
   (ii) Pancreatitis
   (iii) Cholangitis
   (iv) Biliary stricture with cirrhosis
Calot's Triangle:
   (i)   Base: liver
   (ii) Sides: common hepatic duct and cystic duct
   (iii) Contents: cystic artery and right hepatic artery

Pancreas

CAUSES OF ACUTE PANCREATITIS
1. Extrahepatic biliary disease
2. Alcoholism
3. Trauma
4. Postoperative: gastrectomy, biliary surgery, ERCP, afferent loop obstruction
5. Hyperparathyroidism
6. Thiazides, frusemide, steroids
7. Hypothermia
8. Hyperlipidaemia
9. Viral – mumps, Coxsackie
10. Miscellaneous: Polyarteritis nodosa, malignant hypertension

Diagnosis of pancreatitis
Essentially a clinical diagnosis. To be differentiated from conditions with similar clinical and laboratory results, but which require urgent surgery

Clinical features of acute pancreatitis
1. Epigastric pain radiating to back,
2. Vomiting and distension
3. Minimal findings on abdominal examination in sharp contrast with severe symptoms and systemic toxicity in early stages
4. Jaundice, glycosuria, and carpopedal spasm sometimes seen
5. Flank (Grey Turner's) and periumbilical (Cullen's) ecchymosis seen in haemorrhagic pancreatitis

Results of amylase measurement
1. Serum amylase reaches a peak one hour from onset of attack
2. In 30% cases less than 200 Somogyi units – 370 u/l
   30% cases 200–500 Somogyi units – 370–925 u/l
   30% cases more than 500 Somogyi units – 925 u/l.
3. Renal amylase to creatinine clearance ratio rises in acute pancreatitis and sharpens diagnostic accuracy. Should replace simple amylase measurements

Differential diagnosis of acute pancreatitis
These conditions may all be associated with raised serum amylase, but usually normal clearance ratio. Less than 5.0%
1. Penetrating duodenal ulcer
2. Perforated duodenal ulcer
3. Acute cholecystitis
4. Ischaemic bowel
   (i) mesenteric embolus
   (ii) strangulation
5. Myocardial infarction
6. Dissecting aortic aneurysm

Management of acute pancreatitis
1. Nasogastric suction: relief from pain and vomiting
2. Intravenous fluids: to replace retroperitoneal and intra-abdominal fluid sequestration
3. Close monitoring of renal and respiratory function
4. Repeated physical examinations to ensure response to conservative treatment and avoid delayed diagnosis of surgically correctable conditions
5. Check for hypocalcaemia and diabetes
6. Controversial: Trasylol, anticholinergics, glucagon
7. Antibiotics: No evidence that prophylactic antibiotics are of use
8. Diagnosis of cases associated with cholelithiasis – best done by oral cholecystogram at 6 weeks. May get false positives if done earlier. IVC is more useful in early stages/ultrasound
9. Laparotomy: Reserved for cases which do not show signs of improvement, and in which there remains doubt about diagnosis.

Complications of acute pancreatitis
1. Pseudocysts – may become infected and bleed
2. Abscesses
3. Thrombosis or rupture of portal mesenteric vessels
4. Perforation of stomach or duodenum
5. Renal/respiratory failure

Features of chronic pancreatitis
1. May be asymptomatic (calcification on x-ray)
2. Recurrent pain
3. Frequent association with narcotic and alcohol abuse
4. May cause obstructive jaundice
5. Steatorrhoea
6. Diabetes

Management
1. Correction of biliary disease if present
2. Abstinence from alcohol
3. Pancreaticojejunostomy/subtotal pancreatectomy for intractible cases

PANCREATIC TRAUMA
1. May be penetrating/non penetrating
2. Frequently overlooked
3. 80% have elevated amylase
4. Requires laparotomy to exclude major duct injury and provide drainage. Partial pancreatectomy may be required in severe cases

ZOLLINGER-ELLISON SYNDROME
Non ß-islet cell tumour
Consider diagnosis:
1. Fulminant peptic ulcer, with diarrhoea and hypokalaemia
2. Atypical site e.g., 3rd/4th part duodenum or jejunum
3. Rugal hypertrophy
4. 12 hour gastric secretion of 200–300 mEq
5. No augmented response to histamine
6. Elevated gastrin
7. Positive secretin test

60% are malignant
20% are associated with pituitary, parathyroid or adrenocortical adenomas

Treatment. Total gastrectomy

FEATURES OF INSULINOMA
1. 10% malignant, 10% multiple
2. Whipples Triad
   (i) Attacks precipitated by fasting/exercise
   (ii) Fasting blood sugar less than 50 mgm/100 ml
   (iii) Relief of symptoms with glucose

Treatment. Diazoxide for preoperative control of sugar; removal of adenomas; Streptozotocin for functioning metastases

CARCINOMA OF PANCREAS
Poor prognosis is related to late presentation (especially body and tail lesions) viz., 80% have lymph node involvement or liver metastases

Clinical features
1. Unexplained weight loss/malaise
2. Obstructive jaundice
3. 60% have pain, not as severe as biliary colic, and often eased on sitting forwards
4. May have acute onset diabetes
5. 30% have palpable gall bladder

Diagnosis
1. Clinical
2. Barium meal – often unhelpful
3. Scanning and ultrasound – sometimes useful
4. ERCP
5. Arteriography

Treatment
1. Resectable lesions: Pancreaticoduodenectomy (Whipple's)
2. Unresectable lesions:
   (i) Biliary drainage e.g., cholecystojejunostomy
   (ii) Gastric drainage e.g., gastrojejunostomy

Spleen

CAUSES OF SPLENOMEGALY
1. Infections
   (i) Bacterial: typhoid
   (ii) viral: glandular fever
   (iii) parasitic: hydatid
   (iv) protozoal: malaria schistosomiasis
2. Lymphoreticular
   (i) Hodgkins
   (ii) leukaemia (chronic myeloid)
   (iii) polycythaemia
   (iv) myeloid metaplasia
3. Portal hypertension
4. Cysts, abscesses, tumours of spleen
5. Metabolic etc.: amyloid, Gaucher's, Still's, Felty's

INDICATIONS FOR SPLENECTOMY
1. Ruptured spleen
2. Part of other operation e.g., radical gastrectomy
3. Blood disorders: ITP, hereditary spherocytosis
4. Staging of Hodgkin's disease
5. Tumours, cysts

TYPES OF SPLENIC RUPTURE
1. Penetrating trauma
   (i) transabdominal
   (ii) transthoracic
2. Non penetrating trauma
   (i) immediate rupture 90%
   (ii) delayed (3–9 day peak) Most are missed diagnosis
3. Operative trauma
4. Spontaneous rupture—minor trauma to pathologically enlarged or delicate spleen e.g., mononucleosis, pregnancy

Splenic rupture is most common injury following non penetrating abdominal trauma. 30% isolated injury

Presenting features of splenic rupture
1. History of trauma (may be forgotten by patient, especially children)
2. Signs of hypovolamia and tachycardia
3. Epigastric pain and tenderness 30%
4. Pain referred to shoulder (Trendelenburg position)
5. May be minimal/absent initially
6. Flank dullness
7. Leucocytosis occurs early

Investigations which may be used
1. Chest X-ray and abdominal film
2. Peritoneal lavage
3. Arteriography
4. Spleen scan

Most reliable means of diagnosis is repeated clinical examination

X-Ray features suggestive of splenic rupture
1. Elevation and immobility of left diaphragm
2. Increased size of splenic shadow
3. Medial displacement gastric air bubble
4. Depression of splenic flexure
5. Fractured ribs
6. Left Psoas and left renal outline obscured

Complications of splenectomy
1. Haemorrhage
2. Acute dilatation of stomach
3. Left lower lobe collapse
4. Pancreatitis/cyst/abscess
5. Subphrenic abscess
6. Splenic vein thrombosis
7. Septicaemia – risk in children and those with underlying
    immune incompetence
8. Postoperative deep vein thrombosis increased

Hernias

A hernia is the protrusion of a viscus or part of a viscus through an abnormal opening

INCIDENCE:
External abdominal hernias – 5% of population
1. Inguinal 73%
2. Femoral 17%
3. Umbilical 8.5%
4. Rarer forms 1.5%

AETIOLOGY OF HERNIAS
1. Congenital/primary
2. Secondary to raised intra-abdominal pressure
   (i) Cough
   (ii) Constipation
   (iii) Cysts
   (iv) Carcinoma e.g., left colon
   (v) Pregnancy
   (vi) Bladder outlet syndrome
3. Iatrogenic – incisional

PATHOLOGICAL ANATOMY
A hernia consists of:
1. A sac – peritoneal diverticulum
2. Contents include:
   (i) Omentum
   (ii) Bowel: whole/part of circumference
   (iii) Bladder/bladder diverticulum
   (iv) Ovary +/–fallopian tube
   (v) Appendix
   (vi) Meckel's diverticulum
   (vii) Fluid (ascitic)
3. Coverings – the layers of abdominal wall through which the sac passes

Types

Reducible
1. Contents of sac can be completely returned to abdominal cavity
2. Cough impulse present
3. May only be evident on examination of the patient standing
N.B. **Always** examine the patient standing before deciding on the presence of a hernia

Irreducible
1. Contents of sac cannot be completely returned to the peritoneal cavity
2. Cough impulse may/may not be present
3. Painless and non-tender

Strangulated
Most commonly in femoral hernia, (also indirect inguinal, umbilical and obturator). Implies ischaemia of sac contents, which in the case of bowel may become gangrenous and perforate
1. Symptoms
   (i) Sudden onset of pain in a hernia
   (ii) Central colicky abdominal pain
   (iii) Vomiting
   (iv) Absolute constipation of flatus and faeces
   (v) Abdominal distension
   (vi) Within hours, colicky abdominal pain is succeeded by continuous pain which frequently implies ischaemic bowel
2. Signs
   (i) Skin overlying hernia may be red and oedematous
   (ii) Tense, tender, irreducible hernia
   (iii) No cough impulse
   (iv) Bowel sounds increased
3. Differentiate from
   (i) Torsion of testis
   (ii) Tender lymphadenitis

Anatomy of.inguinal canal
A musculo-aponeurotic defect, 1½" long, above and parallel to the inguinal ligament extending from the deep to superficial rings. Transmits the vas deferens in the male and round ligament in the female

Deep Ring
   Lies ½" above the mid-inguinal point in fascia transversalis lateral to inferior epigastric vessels

Superficial Ring
   Lies supero-medial to the pubic tubercle in external oblique aponeurosis

Anterior Wall
   (i) Skin and superficial fascia
   (ii) External oblique aponeurosis
   (iii) Internal oblique laterally

Posterior Wall
   (i) Fascia transversalis
   (ii) Conjoint tendon medially

Above
   Fibres of internal oblique and transversus arching over to form
conjoint tendon

Below
   Inguinal ligament

Anatomy of femoral canal
The most medial compartment of the femoral sheath extending from
the femoral ring to the saphenous opening

1. *Boundaries of the Femoral Ring*
    (i)   Anterior: inguinal ligament
    (ii)   Posterior: ligament of Astley Cooper
    (iii) Medial: Lacunar ligament, sometimes with accessory
           obturator artery
    (iv)   Lateral: femoral vein
    (v)   Contents: Cloquet's lymph node
Femoral hernias are more common in females because the canal is
wider

Inguinal hernia

1. *Indirect type*
    (i)   Transverse the inguinal canal from the deep to the
           superficial rings
    (ii)   May extend into the scrotum
    (iii) Congenital in origin
    (iv)   Liable to strangulate

2. *Direct Type*
    (i)   Protrude through transversalis fascia medial to the
           inferior epigastric vessels (Hesselbach's triangle)
    (ii)   Very rarely strangulate because the neck of the sac is
           wide
    (iii) Always acquired

Femoral hernia
1. Protrude through the femoral canal
2. Most likely to become strangulated with rapid onset of
    gangrene
3. Usually small and therefore easily missed in the obese
4. The sac may contain part of the circumference of a piece of
    bowel resulting in an ischaemic knuckle = Richter's hernia

Features of Richter's hernia
1. Symptoms of gastroenteritis (diarrhoea and abdominal pain)
2. Eventual perforation leading to generalised peritonitis and
    paralytic ileus
3. Late diagnosis, because of easily confused symptoms

Differentiation of inguinal and femoral hernias
1. Inguinal hernia lies above the inguinal ligament
2. Femoral hernia lies below and lateral to inguinal ligament.
    The tip of a large femoral hernia may lies above the inguinal
    ligament due to upward displacement by the attachment of
    the superficial fascia to the saphenous opening
    But:(i)   The neck of the sac lies below the posterior to the
                    inguinal ligament
         (ii)   Invagination of the scrotal skin with the examining
                finger reveals an empty inguinal canal

Umbilical hernia
1. *Exomphalos*
    (i)   Present at birth
    (ii)   Requires surgical repair

2. *Congenital umbilical hernia*
    (i)   Mostly close spontaneously in the first year of life
    (ii)   Surgical repair at 2 years of age if persistent

3. *Umbilical hernia in adults*
    (i)   Especially in obese multiparous women
    (ii)   Narrow neck therefore liable to strangulate
    (iii) Often irreducible because of adhesions within the sac
    (iv)   Contents of sac:
           a. omentum
           b. transverse colon
           c. small bowel
    (v)   Surgical repair – *Mayo's operation:* overlapping of edges
           of the rectus sheath

Epigastric hernia
1. Fatty protrusions through linea alba defect – rarely bowel
2. Pain may be confused with dyspepsia

Obturator hernia
1. Herniation through obturator canal
2. Especially in thin, elderly females
3. Narrow neck therefore liable to strangulate
4. Richter type hernia may occur
5. Pain referred along the medial aspect of the thigh
6. May be felt per rectum/vaginum
7. Easily forgotten cause of intestinal obstruction
8. May present as an 'abscess' on medial aspect of thigh which
    drains faeculent material on incision

Spigelian hernia
1. Herniation via arcuate line into rectus sheath
2. Soft, tender mass to one side of lower abdominal wall

Lumbar hernia

Gluteal hernia

Sciatic hernia

1. All rare
2. Differential diagnosis
   (i) Lipoma
   (ii) Tuberculous abscess
   (iii) Fibrosarcoma

Incisional hernia
  1. Predisposing factors
     (i)   Bad operative technique
     (ii) Cachexia
     (iii) Obesity
     (iv) Steroids
     (v)   Abdominal distension
     (vi) Malignant disease
  2. Begin in the early postoperative period
  3. A sero-sanguinous discharge from a wound sometimes indicates dehiscence and is an indication for careful wound palpation

Treatment of hernias
  1. Preoperative attention to smoking, weight reduction
  2. Investigation and treatment of urinary outlet obstruction or colonic obstruction before hernia repair
  3. Resuscitation for cases presenting with intestinal obstruction
  4. In absence of systemic toxicity analgesics ice packs and gentle manipulation may enable reduction of incarcerated hernia. Oedema then subsides and elective repair is better. There is a risk of reduction 'en masse' i.e., lump disappears but contents remain incarcerated in sac and may become ischaemic. Unrecognised strangulated bowel may also be reduced
  5. Principles of hernia repair
     (i) Identification of sac and contents; mobilisation of sac; reduction of contents; ligation of sac
     (ii) Repair of fascial defect; different methods used; healthy, strong fascial tissue must be opposed without undue tension e.g., inguinal hernias; fascia transversalis to Cooper's ligament or inguinal ligament

Differential diagnosis of a lump in the groin
  1. Hernia
  2. Lymph node
  3. Saphena varix
  4. Lipoma
  5. Femoral aneurysm
  6. Psoas abscess – do not confuse fluctuation with reducibility
  7. Ectopic testis
  8. Hydrocoele of canal of Nuck

Adrenal

CAUSES OF CUSHING'S SYNDROME
1. 90% – adrenal hyperplasia
2. Less commonly – adrenal adenoma/carcinoma, pituitary basophil adenoma
3. Rarely ectopic ACTH e.g., lung carcinoma

Tests for cushing's syndrome
1. Loss of diurnal cortisone rhythm
2. ACTH level decrease in adenoma/carcinoma
3. Metyrapone test results in increase of urinary steroids in hyperplasia/normals
4. Dexamethasone suppression of hyperplasia/normals. (Some adenomas at 8 mg)
5. X-ray of sella turcica
6. Adrenal angiography – tumour localisation
7. Iodocholesterol scan

Treatment of Cushing's syndrome
1. Hyperplasia
   (i) bilateral total adrenalectomy
   (ii) pituitary irradiation given by some because 15% incidence of pituitary adenomas following adrenalectomy
   (iii) maintenance hydrocortisone – 25 mg a.m., 12.5 mg p.m. Most people also give some mineralocorticoid
2. Adenoma/carcinoma
   (i) unilateral adrenalectomy
   (ii) maintenance steroids until suppressed contralateral gland regains function
3. Pituitary adenoma – irradiation

CAUSES OF ACUTE ADRENAL INSUFFICIENCY
1. Rapid withdrawal/failure of absorption of long term steroid therapy – this is most common cause
2. Haemorrhage into adrenals
   (i) Foetal distress
   (ii) Waterhause Friedrichson's syndrome
   (iii) Anticoagulant therapy
   (iv) Pregnancy
   (v) Post venography – adrenal vein thrombosis

Acute adrenal insufficiency does not present with electrolyte abnormalities of Addison's disease, but with
1. Fever
2. Shock
3. Lethargy
4. Nausea

SURGICAL COMPLICATIONS OF STEROID THERAPY
1. Retarded wound healing
2. Pathological fractures
3. Opportunistic postoperative infection, e.g., fungi
4. Upper gastrointestinal ulceration – controversial – may potentiate tendency to form ulcers
5. Pancreatitis
6. Reactivation of TB

Any patient requiring operation who has received long term steroid therapy is best covered perioperatively with supplemental steroids because there is no reliable test of the hypothalamic pituitary axis

ADRENAL MEDULLA
Conditions producing paroxysmal hypertension
1. Anxiety
2. Phaeochromocytoma (90% children and 65% adults have sustained hypertension)
3. Eclampsia
4. Brain tumours
5. Thyroid crisis

Sites for phaeochromocytoma
1. Abdominal
    (i)   adrenal medulla
    (ii)   extra adrenal paraganglia
    (iii) organs of Zuckerkandl
    (iv)   bladder
2. Extra-abdominal
    (i)   brain
    (ii)   neck
    (iii) thorax

Conditions which if present suggest phaeochromocytoma in a hypertensive person
1. Any sort of 'attack'
2. Diabetes mellitus
2. Child without renal disease/coarctation
3   Postural hypotension, excessive sweating, headaches
4. Severe eclampsia
5. Neurofibromatosis
6. Family history or previous history of phaeochromocytoma
7. Recent onset of hypertension with retinopathy

Increased incidence of phaeochromocytoma
1. Hyperparathyroidism
2. Medullary carcinoma of thyroid (Sipple's disease)
3. Von Recklinghausen's
4. Van Hippel Lindau

Preoperative preparation of phaeochromocytoma patient
1. α-Blockers (phentolamine) – to counteract vasoconstriction and hypertension
2. Volume replacement – to correct diminished vascular volume
3. ß-Blockers to slow heart rate and decrease arrhythmias
4. Calcitonin level – exclude medullary thyroid carcinoma
5. Arteriographic localisation
6. Oral cholecystogram to rule out associated gallstones

SUMMARY OF FACTS ABOUT NEUROBLASTOMA
1. Generally in patients less than 5 years old
2. Present commonly as abdominal mass or swelling of head secondary to metastases
3. Very vascular tumours which metastasise widely especially to bone
4. May cause hypertension (associated with raised urinary VMA)
5. Removal followed by radiotherapy can give good results

Urology

KIDNEY AND URETER
Important congenital renal abnormalities
1. Absence of one kidney
2. Pelvic kidney
3. Horseshoe kidney
4. Both kidneys on one side
5. Supernumery renal vessels
6. Polycystic kidneys
7. Duplication of kidney/pelvis/ureter
8. Congenital hydronephrosis

Practical considerations arising from congenital abnormalities
1. Exclude unilateral kidney prior to nephrectomy
2. An abnormal pelvic mass may be renal
3. Ligation of supernumery vessels can cause infarction
4. Polycystic kidneys may be familial, or associated with cysts of liver, pancreas. Also associated with intracerebral berry aneurysms

HAEMATURIA
Causes
1. Infection   40%
2. Tumour   20%
3. Obstruction 15% (prostate)
4. Stone   20%
5. Trauma   5%

Site
1. Kidney   15%
2. Ureter   15%
3. Bladder   40%
4. Prostate 25%
5. Urethra   5%

Don't Forget:
1. Generalised bleeding diatheses
2. Unusual causes: endocarditis, polyartcritis nodosa, malignant hypertension, glomerulonephritis, mitral stenosis, cystic kidneys
3. Tumours are increasingly common after 40 years

Investigation of haematuria
1. Follows careful history and physical examination
2. Urine analysis – RBC's, WBC's, bacteria, casts
3. Plain abdominal film – 80% stones opaque
4. IVP
5. Cystoscopy – gives most information when patient is actively bleeding
6. Angiography and ultrasound for renal masses

CAUSES OF URINARY OBSTRUCTION

1. *Pelvis*
   (i) Congenital pelviureteric junction obstruction
   (ii) Tumour, stone, clot

2. *Ureter*
   (i) Stone/clot
   (ii) Tumour – ureter, bladder, prostate
   (iii) Stricture
   (iv) Ureterocoele
   (v) Aberrant vessels
   (vi) Cancer colon/rectum, cervix
   (vii) Retroperitoneal fibrosis

3. *Urethra*
   (i) Prostate
   (ii) Stricture
   (iii) Foreign bodies
   (iv) Congenital valves

Renal injuries commonly associated with
1. Spleen
2. Liver
3. Pancreas
4. Diaphragm
5. 11th and 12th rib fractures. Fractures of transverse processes

Management of blunt renal injury
1. Bed rest
2. Examination for development of expanding flank haematoma
3. Serial urine examination for clearing of gross haematuria
4. Serial haematocrit, pulse, blood pressure monitoring
95% successfully managed conservatively

Aim of investigation in renal trauma (IVP and arteriogram)
1. Confirm presence of two kidneys
2. Exclude complete renal rupture with perirenal extravasation of blood and urine or avulsion of renal pedicle

Indications for surgery
1. Deteriorating clinical condition e.g., life threatening haemorrhage or expanding flank mass
2. IVP/angiogram evidence of complete rupture or avulsion of kidney
3. Penetrating injuries

CALCULI
Causes of urinary calculi
1. Stasis/infection
   - (i) hydronephrosis
   - (ii) bladder diverticulum
   - (iii) retroprostatic pouch
   - (iv) large residual volume
   - (v) immobility
   - (vi) dehydration e.g., diarrhoea-inflammatory bowel disease—ileostomy
2. Excess of normal constituents
   - (i) hyperparathyroidism – calcium
   - (ii) gout – urate
   - (iii) Crohn's – oxalate, urate, calcium
3. Abnormal urine constituents
   - (i) foreign body (catheter)
   - (ii) epithelial debris – infection

Differential diagnosis of calculus on x-ray
1. Calcified lymph node
2. Gallstones
3. Phleboliths
4. TB
5. Calcified adrenal
6. Pancreatic calcification
7. Radio-opaque pills
8. Calcified fibroids

Management of urinary calculi
90% of calculi less than 4 mm diameter pass spontaneously. Calculi more than 6 mm have less than 20% chance
1. Analgesics
2. High fluid intake
3. Strain urine (stone analysis)
4. Rule out metabolic causes
5. Prophylactic
   - (i) fluid intake
   - (ii) urine pH adjustment

Indications for surgery
1. Increasing size of stone and no movement
2. Stone causing obstruction
3. Repeated and unrelieved colic
4. Recurrent haematuria
5. Urinary infection
6. Large stone

Relief of renal colic can imply passage of stone, but also onset of complete obstruction. Therefore, follow-up IVP essential

Particular sites for impaction
1. Pelviureteric junction
2. Pelvic brim
3. Ureteric orifice

Procedures for removal of calculi
1. Ureteric orifice and lower ureter – stone basket
2. Higher levels – uretero/pyelolithotomy
3. Renal: nephrolithotomy/partial nephrectomy

PREDISPOSING FACTORS FOR URINARY INFECTION
1. Catheterisation
2. Stone
3. Diverticulum
4. Prostatic obstruction
5. Pregnancy
6. Congenital anomalies
7. Vesicouretic reflux
8. Females – short urethra – intercourse

Genitourinary TB
1. Secondary to haematogenous spread from lungs or gut
2. Initially bilateral cortical infection followed by ulceration into collecting system. Results in sterile pyuria, haematuria. No bacteria on gram stain. Some lesions heal, other progress
3. Symptoms of dysuria and frequency follow development of cystitis
4. Fibrosis leads to obstruction at any level
5. Genital TB can exist independently
   (i) epididymitis
   (ii) seminal vesiculitis
   (iii) prostatitis
   (iv) fistula formation

Diagnosis
1. Awareness of disease
2. Appropriate cultures

Treatment
1. Antituberculous drugs
2. Surgery for obstruction – functionless kidney – failed medical treatment

FEATURES OF WILM'S TUMOUR
1. May be present at birth
2. Presents as a loin mass
3. May be bilateral 5%
4. Excision, radiotherapy, chemotherapy can achieve 70% cure rate. Prognosis worse after 2 years of age

ADENOCARCINOMA OF KIDNEY MAY PRESENT AS
1. Haematuria – often painless or pain follows bleeding
2. Abdominal mass
3. Loin pain
4. Pathological fracture
5. Anaemia, weight loss, fever of unknown origin
6. Polycythaemia 4%
7. Acute onset left varicocoele
8. Endocrine syndromes

TUMOURS OF RENAL PELVIS
1. Transitional cell lesions
   (i)   non invasive
   (ii)   invasive
2. Squamous cell carcinoma following metaplasia; bleed less; present later; worse prognosis

Treatment of renal tumours
1. Adenocarcinoma
   (i)   nephrectomy
   (ii)   removal of solitary metastases
   (iii)   some advocate preoperative irradiation
2. Transitional and squamous lesions
   (i)   nephroureterectomy
   (ii)   local excision rarely e.g., if solitary kidney

BLADDER
Complications associated with ectopia vesicae
1. Urinary infection and pyelonephritis
2. Epispadias
3. Inguinal hernia
4. Carcinoma of bladder remnant
5. Pelvic bone abnormalities – waddling gait

Rupture of the bladder
1. A full bladder is more prone to rupture
2. Can be easily missed in presence of more obvious injuries
3. Heavy drinkers are at special risk

Causes of extraperitoneal rupture
1. Pelvic fracture
2. Iatrogenic – in herniorrhaphy/hysterectomy

Causes of intraperitoneal rupture
1. Blunt trauma to abdominal wall
2. Missile injuries
3. Instrumentation

Principles of treatment
1. Repair bladder defect
2. Drain retropubic space
3. Divert urine with urethral or suprapubic catheter

Complications of bladder diverticula
(Double Micturition)
1. Infection
2. Calculus formation
3. Malignant change
4. Obstruction of adjacent ureter
5. Rupture

Causes of bladder calculus
1. Foreign bodies – catheter
2. Stasis/infection., prostate, stricture, diverticulum

Symptoms of bladder calculus
1. Trigone irritation/pain – sitting, standing, on stairs
2. Haematuria
3. Infection

Aetiology of bladder tumours
1. ß-naphthylamine
2. Smoking
3. Saccharin?
4. Schistosomiasis (Squamous cell carcinoma)

Types of bladder tumours
1. Transitional cell papilloma – 80% non invasive (i.e., basement membrane intact) tend to be multiple and recurrent. 25% become invasive

Stages of invasive transitional cell carcinoma

Stage A:	Invasion of submucosa
Stage B_1:	Invasion of superficial muscle layer
Stage B_2:	Invasion of deep muscle layer
Stage C:	Invasion of perivesical adventitia and lymphatics
Stage D:	Distant metastases or fixed tumour

Prognosis is most related to depth of invasion and differentiation

Bladder may be involved by tumours from
1. Rectum
2. Uterus
3. Ovary
4. Prostate
5. (Endometriosis)

Clinical features
1. Painless haematuria
2. Clot retention
3. Obstruction of adjacent ureter
4. Sometimes frequency and dysuria

Investigation
1. Urinalysis (RBC's, tumour cells)
2. IVP
3. Cystoscopy – biopsy
4. Bimanual examination under anaesthesia. Detect extension beyond bladder

Treatment: depends on
1. Age and general condition of patient
2. Depth of invasion
3. Site in bladder

Non invasive papilloma and Stage A carcinoma
1. Endoscopic resection
2. Regular follow-up cystoscopy

B_1
Controversial – some use endoscopic resection, others total cystectomy with/without radiotherapy
Partial cystectomy with 2 cm margin of normal tissue may be used for lesions in vault of bladder
B_2/C
1. Total cystectomy often with preoperative irradiation
2. Ileal loop

D. Symptomatic treatment e.g. irradiation

Principles in managing neurogenic bladder
1. Catheter drainage with closed irrigation system until cystometry shows return of reflex activity. Intermittent catheterisation increasingly popular
2. Clean external meatus to discourage ascending infection
3. Increase fluid intake to obtain high urine output (2 l/day)
4. Acidify urine with ascorbic acid to discourage stone formation
5. Low calcium diet if urinary calcium excretion is more than 300 mg/day
6. Regular urine cultures and appropriate antibotics

PROSTATE

Typical symptoms of prostatic disease
1. Poor intermittent stream – worse on straining
2. Frequency urgency, dysuria and nocturia
3. Haematuria
4. Retention of urine (remember as cause of confusion in elderly)
5. Vague complaints of ill health – uraemia

Complications of prostatic disease
1. Bladder hypertrophy and formation of diverticulae
2. Urinary infection – often related to catheterisation
3. Bladder calculi
4. Hydronephrosis and renal failure
5. Haemorrhoids, hernias, rectal prolapse from straining
6. Effects of metastases e.g., bone

Typical findings on rectal examination
1. Benign enlargement chiefly involves middle and lateral lobes – smooth enlargement with well defined central sulcus. Considerable middle lobe enlargement can occur in absence of palpable mass
2. Malignant disease chiefly affects posterior lobe – craggy mass ill defined and hard with obliteration of sulcus. Early cases felt as a nodule

Other causes of induration on rectal examination
1. Prostatitis
2. Prostatic calculi
3. Extension of rectal/bladder tumour
4. TB

Investigation of prostatic disease
1. Blood: Assess renal function
   (i) Bone marrow (Secondaries)
   (ii) Acid phosphatase increased in 70% cases
2. IVP:
   (i) Trabeculation/diverticulae
   (ii) Calculi
   (iii) Hydronephrosis
   (iv) Smooth filling defect at base
   (v) Residual urine on post micturition film
3. Skeletal views for osteoblastic metastases. Prostatic carcinoma spreads to vertebral veins and skeleton
4. Needle biopsy of nodules (50% are malignant)

Indications for elective treatment of benign disease
1. Marked symptoms
2. Large residual volume
3. Diverticula
4. Dilated ureters
5. Calculi
6. Persistent urinary infection

Treatment of benign disease
1. Open prostatectomy:
   (i)   For very large glands
   (ii) If diverticulae require treatment in addition
2. Transurethral resection

Treatment of prostatic carcinoma
1. Very early disease e.g. nodule
   (i)   Staging   bone marrow
                   lymphangiogram
                   liver scan
                   lung tomograms
   (ii) Irradiation
2. Advanced disease
   (i)   Orchidectomy/Oestrogens
   (ii)   Transurethral resection when oestrogens fail to relieve obstruction
   (iii) Irradiation of painful metastases
   (iv)   Hypophysectomy/Adrenalectomy after relapse on oestrogens

Complications of Stilboestrol
1. Fluid retention
2. Thrombosis
3. Gynaecomastia

Causes of urinary retention

1. *Local*
   (i)   Prostatic disease
   (ii)   Stricture
   (iii) Trauma
   (iv)   Stone
   (v)   Blood clot
   (vi)   Meatal ulcer
   (vii) Urethritis
   (viii) Prostatitis/abscess
2. *Pelvis*
   (i)   Tumour
   (ii)   Pregnant uterus

3. *Neurological*
   (i)   Diabetes
   (ii) Spinal cord compression – tumour – disc
   (iii) Tabes

4. *Drugs*
   Probanthene

5. *General*
   Postoperative

URETHRA
Urethral valves
A readily treatable and easily forgotten cause of uraemia,
hypertension and recurrent urinary infection in children

Rupture of bulbous urethra
1. Follows direct blow/rough instrumentation
2. Patient has perineal pain and haematoma
3. May have blood on meatus

Rupture of membranous urethra
1. Usually associated with pelvic fracture
2. On rectal examination prostatic displacement may be felt with
   complete tears

Management
1. In suspected cases see if patient can void
2. Obtain expert help and do not catheterise
3. Urethrogram to show site and extent of damage
4. Operative treatment
   (i)   Membranous ruptures:
         a. Drain periprostatic and perivesical spaces
         b. Divert urine with suprapubic catheter
         c. Re-establish urethral continuity by antegrade passage
            of catheter from bladder to severed proximal end, and
            'railroad' a catheter from distal end through to
            bladder. Balloon is inflated and traction approximates
            severed ends for 3 weeks
   (ii) bulbous ruptures:
         a. Divert urine with suprapubic drain
         b. Open repair of severed ends – at time or later
Postoperative dilatation is necessary to prevent strictures

Causes of urethral strictures
1. Trauma – rupture, surgery, catheter
2. Infective – gonorrhoea, TB

Complications of stricture
1. From straining at micturition–piles, hernia, rectal prolapse
2. Proximal urethritis
3. Periurethritis
4. Periurethral abscess and fistula
5. Prostatitis
6. Epididymitis
7. Cystitis
8. Pyelonephritis
9. Hydronephrosis

Treatment
Repeat dilatations to avoid surgery which has poor results

Causes of acute urethritis
1. Gonorrhoea
2. Trichomonas
3. Mimae
4. Reiter's syndrome (arthritis, conjunctivitis, urethritis)

Complications of gonorrhoea
(Always exclude concomittant syphillis)
1. Urethral stricture
2. Prostatitis
3. Tubo ovarian abscess, salpingitis, peritonitis
4. Ectopic pregnancy
5. Sterility
6. Arthritis – polyarticular in 80%
7. Tenosynovitis
8. Bursitis
9. Ophthalmitis
10. Perihepatitis
11. Endocarditis

TESTIS
Classification of undescended testis

1. *Rectractile*
Scrotal skin is normally developed. After crouching, a warm bath, or gentle manipulation, normal position can be obtained

2. *Ectopic*
Descent to an abnormal site e.g.,
 (i) Superficial inguinal pouch
 (ii) Groin
 (iii) Perineum
 (iv) Root penis
 (v) Femoral triangle

3. *Maldescended*
Lies anywhere in normal descent line from abdominal wall to top of scrotum

Complications of ectopic/maldescended testis
1. Infertility – if bilateral
2. Twenty fold increase in malignancy
3. Increased incidence of trauma
4. Increased incidence of torsion
5. Can be associated with hernia 70%
6. Can be associated with other genito-urinary abnormalities

Treatment
To provide maximum chance of normal maturation treat by 5–6 years of age. Not known if treatment decreases incidence of malignancy

Operation
Orchidopexy – mobilization of testicle, after identification. Biopsy and secure in scrotum. Repair associated hernia.
Chromatin test and IVP should be done in bilateral cases
Chromatin test and IVP should be done

Examination of scrotal swelling
1. Can your fingers get above swelling? i.e., differentiate from hernia
2. Is swelling
   (i)   Solid/cystic (transilluminate)
   (ii) 'hot'/'cold'
3. Do rectal examination
   (i)   Tender prostate – infection
   (ii) Thickened seminal vesicles ('TB')
   (iii) Enlarged lymph nodes – malignancy
4. Examine neck and abdomen for enlarged nodes
5. Always examine patient lying and standing

Differential diagnosis of scrotal swellings

	Hot	Cold
Solid	Torsion	Tumour
	Epididymitis	TB
	orchitis (mumps)	
Cystic	Infected hydrocoele	Hydrocoele
		Epididymal cyst

'Bag of worms' – varicocoele

A Hydrocoele. May be secondary to an underlying testicular tumour. Therefore, aspirate and then carefully palpate testicle

An Acute Epididymitis that does not show signs of resolution within three weeks of antibiotic therapy should be explored to exclude a missed tumour

Torsion. Occurs in 15–25 year age group most often, presenting as a painful testis and lower abdominal pain with nausea/vomiting. Commonly misdiagnosed as epididymitis. Doppler and isotope scanning can be used. Any young person with an acutely painful testicle should be explored if there is doubt about the diagnosis. Following torsion the testis becomes nonviable in about 4 hours. The other testis should be secured as it is at risk of undergoing torsion subsequently

Suspect a testicular tumour with
1.   Painless lump – not necessarily
2.   Lymphadenopathy
3.   Abdominal mass
4.   Secondary hydrocoele
5.   Gynaecomastia
6.   History of undescended testicle
7.   Any young patient with scrotal swelling

Classification and spread

	Incidence	Age	Spread
Seminoma	60%	30–40 years	Lymphatic
Teratoma	40%	20–30 years	Bloodstream

Treatment
1.   Prove diagnosis – explore via inguinal incision and control cord structures to avoid dissemination of tumour during handling
2.   Radical orchidectomy if tumour found
3.   Stage disease – chest X-ray, IVP, lymphangiogram
4.   Radiotherapy to retroperitoneal, mediastinal and cervical nodes
5.   Chemotherapy for disseminated disease

Nervous system

CAUSES OF INTRACRANIAL MASS
1. Tumour
2. Haematoma
3. Abscess
4. Hydatid, TB, Gumma – rare

FEATURES OF RAISED INTRACRANIAL PRESSURE
1. Headache – worse in morning, and coughing
2. Vomiting – often without nausea
3. Blurred vision
4. Mental deterioration and drowsiness.
5. Increased head circumference – in infants
6. Occurs early with posterior fossa and midline lesions; late with frontal lesions
7. Papilloedema may not be present

Mechanism of increased CSF pressure
1. Mass effect within rigid cranium
2. Surrounding oedema
3. Block to circulation of CSF

CLASSIFICATION OF TUMOURS
1. Glioma – most common
   (i) Astrocytoma 80%
   (ii) Medulloblastoma
   (iii) Oligodentroglioma
   (iv) Ependymoma
2. Meningioma
3. Neurilemmoma – acoustic neuroma
4. Pituitary tumours
5. Metastases
6. Rarer – craniopharyngioma, dermoids, vascular tumours

Clinical features suggesting a tumour
1. Progressive focal neurological deficit
2. Late onset epilepsy
3. Dementia
4. Symptoms of raised intracranial pressure
5. History of primary carcinoma e.g., bronchus/kidney

In children 70% are infratentorial
In adults 70% are supratentorial

Common sites for meningiomas
1. Sphenoid ridge
2. Olfactory groove
3. Suprasellar region
4. Vault
5. Falx
6. Spinal canal

Types of pituitary tumour
1. Chromophobe – most common, some secrete prolactin
2. Eosinophil adenoma – gigantism/acromegaly
3. Basophil adenoma – Cushing's

Complications of pituitary tumours
1. Bitemporal hemianopia
2. Hypopituitarism
3. Diabetes insipidus
4. Hormonal secretion, e.g., Cushing's syndrome, Acromegaly

Features of acoustic neuroma
1. VIII nerve palsy – deafness tinnitus, vertigo
2. VII nerve palsy – facial weakness, unilateral taste loss
3. V nerve palsy – facial numbness, loss of corneal reflex
4. IX, X, nerve palsy – dysphagia, hoarseness
5. Cerebellar syndrome
6. Raised intracranial pressure

Investigation of brain tumours
1. CAT/EMI scanning is rapidly superceding all other methods
2. Chest X-ray – essential since high number of bronchial carcinomas present with cerebral secondaries
3. Skull X-ray may show
   (i) Calcification in
      a. tumour – craniopharyngioma; oligodendrogliomas
      b. vascular anomalies
      c. (TB), toxoplasmosis
   (ii) Hyperostosis – meningioma
   (iii) Shift of pineal
   (iv) Erosion of the sella turcica
   (v) Widening of sutures in infants
4. Angiography – tumour blush/vessel displacement
5. Air encephalogram/ventriculogram. Being done less frequently
6. EEG

Summary of treatment
1. Removal of benign lesions
2. Partial removal of malignant lesions for biopsy/decompression
   Mainstay of treatment is irradiation and steroids
3. Shunts for hydrocephalus
4. Chemotherapy – under trial

CAUSES OF CEREBRAL ABSCESS
1. Spread from
    (i)   Ear infection – cerebellum and temporal lobe
    (ii) Sinus infection – e.g., Frontal lobe
2. Blood spread. Bronchiectasis, cyanotic congenital heart
    disease. May be multiple
3. Penetrating trauma – rare today

Clinical features of cerebral abscess
1. Usually presents as a space occupying lesion in a toxic
    patient
2. May have insidious or rapid onset
3. Systemic toxicity may be absent
4. Localising signs may be absent and late in onset
5. May present years after initiating infection

Management of cerebral abscess
1. Aspiration
2. Systemic and local antibiotics
3   Monitoring of abscess size using CAT/EMI scan
4. Anticonvulsants
5. Late excision of scar sometimes stops seizures

COMMON SITES FOR INTRACRANIAL ANEURYSMS
1. Internal carotid 35%
2. Anterior cerebral 35%
3. Middle cerebral 20%
4. Vertebrobasilar 10%
5. Multiple 20%

Complications of aneurysms
1. Haemorrhage – subarachnoid/intracerebral
    (i)   High initial mortality
    (ii) Recurrent bleed peak incidence at 7 to 12 days carries
          40% mortality. Declines sharply after six weeks

Management
            a. Bed rest
            b. EACA
            c. Angiography for cases with good neurological
                prognosis, before the time of maximum recurrent
                bleeding
            d. Surgery if possible
2. Pressure – Prior to rupture local pressure effect can cause
    headache, cranial nerve palsy, e.g., III

Features of angiomas
1. May cause focal epilepsy
2. Headaches
3. Progressive neurological deficit
50% have bruit

IMMEDIATE MANAGEMENT OF HEAD INJURY
1. Ensure adequate airway
2. Control haemorrhage e.g., scalp wounds
3. Maintain circulation
4. Obtain baseline neurological function
5. Evaluate other injuries
6. Immobilise neck if injury suspected

Cervical spine injuries are easily missed

Hypotension, tachycardia and shock are due to some cause other than the head injury e.g., hidden chest/abdominal trauma

Neurological evaluation of head injury
1. Accurate documentation of level of consciousness and length of amnesia in specific terms; complete physical examination
2. Skull X-rays may show
   (i)   Pineal shift
   (ii) Fracture – e.g., over middle meningeal artery
   (iii) Air in skull
   (iv) Foreign body
3. Cross table lateral cervical spine x-ray with shoulders pulled down for clear view of C_1 – T_1 alignment – in cases where spinal injury suspected

Complications of head injury – about 10%
1. Acute haemorrhage: Any diminution in level of consciousness is assumed to be due to pressure from haematoma. However, other causes viz – airway obstruction, intraperitoneal bleeding, must be excluded

Diminished consciousness level may be followed by
   (i)   Unilateral dilation of pupil and sluggish light reflex
   (ii) Systolic hypertension
   (iii) Bradycardia

Management of haemorrhage
   Call for neurosurgical help
   (i)   Intubate
   (ii) I.V. mannitol 1 g/Kg
   (iii) Catheterise
   (iv) Burr holes on side of dilated pupil
         In practice there is seldom the need for burr holes, to be done in casualty department. In cases of slower bleeds mannitol may control situation long enough to do an arteriogram or CAT scan to help localise lesion, and enable more accurate siting of craniotomy in sterile environment
   (v)   Dexamethasone
2. Skull fracture
   (i)   May be compound via skin, nose/ear. Patients with CSF leaks may require prophylactic antibiotics (controversial). Wounds-debrided, closed
   (ii) Depressed fragments may require elevation if depressed more than 1 cm, lie over motor area, fragment is sharp

3. Meningitis – may follow compound fractures
4. Diabetes insipidus/inappropriate ADH release from pituitary damage
5. Hyperpyrexia – hypothalamic injury
6. Convulsions – especially if long period of unconsciousness
7. Chronic subdural haematoma – in very young and elderly. Trivial injury may present weeks later with fluctuating level of consciousness.
   Easy to miss
8. Hydrocephalus – usually self limiting but may require shunting
9. Psychological problems
   (i)   Personality change
   (ii) Mood – depression
   (iii) Loss of memory, headaches, fatigue
10. Anosmia
11. Long term severe cases require skin, bowel, catheter, nutritional care

TYPES OF SPINA BIFIDA

1) *Spina Bifida Occulta*. In 20% population. Usually asymptomatic Skin dimple, hairtuft, or angioma may mark site in lumbar area. Can be associated with bony spur in spinal canal, causing enuresis, foot drop, bachache. Treatable by excision of spur

2) *Dermal Sinus Tract*. May be hidden by hair. Cause of recurrent meningitis with mixed flora. Treatment – excise

3) *Meningocoele*. Meninges protrude – should be excised and strong tissue brought over deficit to prevent ulceration. No neurological defect

4) *Myelomeningocoele and Myelocoele*. (i) Mixed upper and lower motor neurone deficit (ii) Sphincter disturbance (iii) Scoliosis, congenital dislocation hips, talipes common (iv) Nearly all have hydrocephalus from Arnold Chiari malformation

Management

1. Conservative for those with poor prognosis
   (i)   Flaccidity
   (ii) Severe hydrocephalus
   (iii) Multiple anomalies
2. Surgery
   (i)   Closure of defect within first few hours of life to prevent infection
   (ii) Shunt for hydrocephalus if it develops
3. Orthopaedic and urological procedures later
4. Physiotherapy and special training

COMPLICATIONS OF SPINAL INJURIES

1. *Transection of cord.* Signs depend on level and degree of transection
   1. Include
      - (i)   initial flaccid paralysis
      - (ii)   initial areflexia, later hypereflexia
      - (iii) sensory loss
      - (iv) sphincter denervation – retention, impaction
      - (v)   hypotension – sympathectomy
      - (iv) priapism – useful diagnostic sign

2 *Cauda Equina Injury.* Below L_1; lower motor neurone lesion. Injury is more common at junction of mobile and fixed portions of vertebral column e.g., lower cervical – upper and lower lumbar areas

Management of spinal cord injuries
1. Immobilisation
   - (i)   Four poster collar
   - (ii)   Crutchfield tongs
   - (iii) Stryker frame
2. Decompression. Laminectomy in cases with spinal canal block indicated by progressive signs of compression and myelography. Surgery is rarely required
3. In paraplegics care of
   - (i)   Skin – pressure areas
   - (ii)   Bladder – (see p. 114)
   - (iii) Bowels, enemas, etc.
   - (iv) Internal fixation of unstable vertebral fractures

4. Rehabilitation
Patients with spinal injuries may not have local pain and tenderness, therefore high index of suspicion is required to avoid causing further injury by failure to immobilise (fracture dislocations may reduce spontaneously, and x-rays may not show injury initially). If in doubt immobilise

COMMON SITES FOR PROLAPSED INTERVERTEBRAL DISCS
Usually occur posterolaterally

L_4–5 ⎞	affects L_5	root
80%		
L_5–S_1 ⎠	affects S_1	root
C_5–6 ⎞	affects C_6	root
19%		
C_6–7 ⎠	affects C_7	root

General features
1. Pain
   (i)   Cervical disc – arm pain – interscapular area
   (ii) Lumbar – sciatica – brought on by straight leg raising
2. Weakness and atrophy of muscles
3. Diminished reflexes
4. Sensory loss
5. Local paravertebral muscle spasm and loss of lordosis

Central prolapse of disc
1. Sudden paralysis
2. Sphincter disorder
3. Bilateral sciatica

Localising signs
1. L_5
   (i)   Weakness of Ext Hallucis Longus
   (ii) Decreased sensation dorsum of foot
2. S_1
   (i)   Weakness of plantar flexion
   (ii) Ankle reflex loss
   (iii) Sensation decreased over lateral side of foot
3. C_6
   (i)   Weak biceps and wrist extensors
   (ii) Loss of biceps and brachioradialis reflex
   (iii) Sensory loss on thumb
4. C_7
   (i)   Weak triceps
   (ii) Triceps reflex decreased
   (iii) Sensory loss over middle finger

Indications for surgery of lumbar disc prolapse
1. Central prolapse – emergency
2. Unremitting symptoms following conservative treatment, e.g. bed rest, traction
3. Severe neurological disturbance

Differential diagnosis of sciatica
1. Spinal tumour – primary/secondary
2. Intermittent claudication
3. Osteoarthrosis
4. Rectal and prostatic carcinoma
5. Claudication of the cauda equina
Rectal examination must be done in all cases of sciatica

Causes and features of extradural spinal abscess
1. Septicaemia
2. Osteomyelitis of spine
3. Epidural anaesthetic

Presents as pain, tenderness, fever, paralysis

Causes of spinal cord compression
1. Extradural
   (i) Metastases to spine
   (ii) Lymphoma, myeloma
   (iii) Disc, vertebral collapse, spondylosis
   (iv) TB, abscess
   (v) Haematoma
2. Intradural extramedullary
   (i) Meningioma }
   (ii) Neurofibroma } vast majority
   (iii) Arachnoid cyst, etc. rare
3. Intramedullary
   (i) Glioma
   (ii) Syringo/haematomyelia

Causes of hydrocephalus
1. Congenital
   (i) Chiari malformation
   (ii) Aqueduct stenosis
   (iii) Obstructed foramina of Magendie and Luscha
2. Acquired
   (i) Subarachnoid haemorrhage
   (ii) Meningitis
   (iii) Tumour

PERIPHERAL NERVE INJURIES
Classification of nerve injuries
1. Neurapraxia
   (i) Axon and sheath intact
   (ii) Compression/stretch common causes
   (iii) Good prognosis
2. Axonotmesis
   (i) Sheath intact
   (ii) Axonal disruption
   (iii) Axons regenerate at rate of 1mm/day. Sensory function usually returns well. If site of injury is greater than 40 cm from denervated muscle, then permanent muscle atrophy will occur by the time reinnervation takes place
3. Neurotmesis
   Sheath and axonal disruption. Prognosis better for pure sensory/motor nerves. In mixed nerves cross innervation occurs. Accurate apposition of severed ends is key factor

Causes of peripheral nerve injuries
1. Pressure e.g., tourniquet, crutch, plaster cast
2. Closed/open injuries e.g., dislocations, stab wounds

Management of peripheral nerve injuries
1. Maintain position of function
2. Active/passive range of motion
3. Surgery for neurotmesis with microscopic apposition
   (i)   Immediate for clean wounds
   (ii) Delayed for contaminated wounds
Transposition/nerve interposition grafts sometimes required.
Tendon transfer for increase of function. Arthrodesis for unstable joints

Specific peripheral nerve injuries.

1. Brachial plexus

Erb's paralysis. C_5 C_6 injury after the head is forced away from the shoulder e.g., obstetric injury
   (i)   Motor deficit; loss of abduction and lateral rotation of shoulder; loss of flexion and supination of elbow; weakness of wrist extension
   (ii) Sensory deficit; upper outer shoulder

Klumpke's paralysis. T_1 e.g. cervical rib, Pancoast tumour
   (i)   Motor deficit; loss of intrinsic muscles of the hand, except supplied by the Median nerve (Abductor, Opponens, and Fl. Poll. Brevis, and lateral two lumbricals)
   (ii) Sensory deficit; Medial two fingers and medial forearm.
   (iii) Horner's syndrome may be present

2. Radial nerve. e.g., crutch palsy, fracture of humerus (spiral groove).
   (i)   Motor deficit; wrist drop – due to wrist extensor paralysis; nerve injury in the axilla can weaken triceps
   (ii) Sensory deficit; very small area between dorsum of thumb and index

3. Median nerve. e.g., elbow fractures, wrist lacerations; carpal tunnel syndrome.
   (i)   Motor deficit; **Wrist level.** Loss of thenar muscles except adductor pollicis. Detected clinically by loss of abduction of the thumb. **Elbow level** Loss of pronators of the forearm and digital flexors (except Fl.C. Ulnaris and Fl.D. Profundus to ring and little fingers) in addition to thenar muscle loss as above
   (ii) Sensory deficit; **Wrist level** Thumb and lateral two and half fingers—palmar aspects. **Elbow level** Radial 2/3 of palm as well as above

4. *Ulnar nerve.* e.g., elbow or wrist injury
  (i)   Motor deficit. **Wrist level** Loss of all the intrinsic muscles of the hand except those supplied by the Median nerve (see above). **Elbow level** Loss of Fl.C. Ulnaris and Fl.D. Profundus to ring and little fingers as well as the above
  (ii) Sensory deficit **Wrist level** medial 1 ½ fingers. **Elbow level** medial palm as well as above

5. *Sciatic nerve* e.g., penetrating wound, posterior dislocation of hip
  (i)   Motor deficit. Foot drop; loss of all movement below knee level; paralysis of the hamstrings
  (ii) Sensory deficit. below knee except for the area medially supplied by long saphenous nerve

6. *Common Peroneal Nerve.* e.g., plaster cast causing pressure at point where the nerve winds round the neck of the fibula
  (i)   Motor deficit; foot drop; loss of eversion
  (ii) Sensory deficit; anterior and lateral aspect of foot

Orthopaedics

CAUSES OF LOW BACK PAIN
1. Trauma e.g.,
    (i)   Sprain
    (ii) Disc prolapse
    (iii) Fracture
2. Inflammatory e.g.,
    (i)   Rheumatoid arthritis
    (ii) Ankylosing spondylitis
3. Degenerative e.g.,
    (i)   Osteoarthritis
    (ii) Disc prolapse
    (iii) Osteoporosis
4. Neoplastic e.g., Primary/secondary tumours
5. Infections e.g.,
    (i)   TB
    (ii) Osteomyelitis
6. Functional e.g.,
    (i)   Postural
    (ii) Pregnancy
    (iii) Unequal leg length
7. Structural e.g.,
    (i)   Spondylosis
    (ii) Spondylolisthesis
    (iii) Sacralisation of L_5

Use of surgery in cerebral palsy
1. Tendon lengthening to weaken spastic muscles
2. Tendon transposition to improve joint function
3. Arthrodesis to stabilise deformed/contracted joints
4. Osteotomy to correct deformity/limb length

Causes of scoliosis
1. Postural
2. Structural
    (i)   Idiopathic – 90%
    (ii) Osteopathic e.g., hemivertebrae
    (iii) Myopathic e.g., dystrophies
    (iv) Neuropathic e.g., polio
    (v)   Iatrogenic e.g., chest surgery, irradiation

Types of contracture
1. Congenital e.g., club foot
2. Acquired
    (i)   Muscle e.g., Volkmann's, polio
    (ii) Fascia e.g., Dupuytren's
    (iii) Joint e.g., rheumatoid arthritis
    (iv) Skin e.g., burns

CLINICAL FEATURES OF FRACTURES
1. Pain and local tenderness
2. Swelling
3. Bruising
4. Deformity
5. Instability
6. Crepitus

Management of fractures
1. General assessment of whole patient
2. Assessment of fracture
   (i) Vascular injury e.g., supracondylar fractures and brachial artery
   (ii) Nerve injury e.g., humeral fractures and radial nerve
   (iii) Skin viability or compound fracture
   (iv) X-rays – correlate with physical findings
3. Temporary splinting
   (i) Minimises further soft tissue injury
   (ii) Reduces bleeding
   (iii) Reduces pain
4. Reduction of fracture – closed/open
5. Immobilisation – internal fixation or external cast/traction
6. Maintenance of function – physiotherapy
7. Rehabilitation
8. Prevention and treatment of complications
   (i) Shock e.g., pelvic fractures
   (ii) Pulmonary embolus – anticoagulation of immobilised patients
   (iii) Fat embolism – (see p. 19)
   (iv) Cast pressure – avoid local pressure, split casts until swelling subsides
   (v) Pressure sores – good nursing
   (vi) Renal calculi – maintain high fluid intake
   (vii) 'Cast syndrome' e.g., paralytic ileus, gastric dilatation

Indications for open reduction and internal fixation
1. Associated major vessel injury
2. To facilitate soft tissue coverage
3. Pathological fractures
4. Multiple fractures
5. Special sites e.g., neck of femur

Management of compound fractures
Aim is to prevent infection
1. Early debridement
2. Antibiotics
3. Immobilisation
4. Obtain soft tissue cover of
   (i)   Bone
   (ii) Tendons
   (iii) Nerve
5. Leave skin open in contaminated cases

Signs of union
1. Clinical
   (i)   No tenderness
   (ii) No abnormal movement
   (iii) No pain on stress
2. Radiological – lags behind clinical union by weeks or months

Causes of nonunion
1. Excess soft tissue destruction
   (i)   at time of injury
   (ii) during open reduction
2. Certain fractures – poor vascularity e.g.,
   (i)   Neck of femur
   (ii) Scaphoid
   (iii) Talus
3. Inadequate immobilisation
4. Soft tissue interposition between fragments
5. Infection
6. Over distraction of fracture
7. Deficiency states e.g., scurvy

Causes of pathological fractures
Fracture in abnormal bone weakened by previous disease
1. Congenital e.g., osteogenesis imperfecta
2. Degenerative e.g., osteoporosis
3. Neoplastic e.g., primary/secondary tumours/cysts
4. Metabolic e.g.,
   (i)   Steroids
   (ii) Paget's
   (iii) Hyperparathyroidism
   (iv) Scurvy

Features of fractures in children
1. Heal rapidly
2. Nonunion is extremely rare
3. Increased limb length may result from stimulation of epiphyses
4. Epiphyseal fractures may lead to growth impairment
5. Open reduction usually contraindicated except in elbow and hip fractures

Features of osteogenic sarcoma

1. *Age*
   (i)   Most common in second decade
   (ii) In elderly secondary to Paget's disease

2. *Site*
   (i)   Lower femur 50%
   (ii) Upper tibia 20%
   (iii) Humerus 10%

3. *Clinical features*
   (i)   Pain – especially at night
   (ii) Bronchitis/pneumonia – lung metastases
   (iii) Local swelling
   (iv) Pathological fracture

4. *X-ray*
   (i)   Osteolytic/osteosclerotic lesion
   (ii) Sun-ray appearance – spicules of new bone
   (iii) Codman's triangle – periosteal elevation

5. *Spread*
   Early bloodstream spread to lungs

6. *Treatment*
   (i)   Early disease – amputation
   (ii) Advanced disease – radiotherapy and chemotherapy

Management of metastases to bone
1. Analgesics
2. Prophylactic intramedullary pinning – femur, humerus
3. Irradiation
4. Hormones e.g., prostate, breast
5. Treat hypercalcaemia
6. Laminectomy and cord decompression

Important causes of hip pain in children
1. Irritable hip – toxic synovitis
2. Perthe's
3. Slipped femoral
4. Infections – TB and pyogenic

Examination of a joint
1. Inspect: e.g., swelling, position, erythema, gait
2. Palpate:
   (i) Temp
   (ii) Effusion
   (iii) Active motion
   (iv) Passive motion
   (v) Stability
3. Specific tests: e.g., Thomas', Trendelenberg, McMurray
4. Examine both sides
5. Assess patient's general health and involvement of other joints

Features of gonococcal arthritis
1. More common in females
2. Initially a migratory polyarthritis which eventually localises in one or two joints especially knee, wrist, elbow
3. Diagnosis by aspiration and culture of joint effusion
4. Penicillin is antibiotic of choice

Uses of surgery in rheumatoid arthritis
When rest and anti-inflammatory drugs fail
1. Synovectomy – before significant collapse/narrowing of joint space
2. Arthrodesis/arthroplasty for unstable or severely incapacitating joints
3. Tendon repair for ruptured tendons
4. Median nerve decompression for carpal tunnel syndrome

Uses of surgery in osteoarthritis
1. Osteotomy for pain
   (i) Femoral osteotomy – relieves hip pain
   (ii) Proximal tibial osteotomy – knee pain
2. Arthroplasty: e.g., cup arthroplasty
3. Femoral head replacement
4. Total hip replacement

Complications of joint replacement
1. Infection
2. Loosening
3. Dislocation
4. Thrombophlebitis especially hip

Indications for amputation
1. Dead extremity e.g., peripheral vascular disease
2. Deadly extremity
   (i) Tumour
   (ii) Extensive infection
3. Dead useless extremity
   (i) Extensive trauma
   (ii) Paralysis

Suggestions for further reading

Bailey, H. & Love, R.J.M. (1977)
A Short Practice of Surgery London: Lewis

Current Problems in Clinical Surgery.
(A periodical published by Year Book Medical, Chicago.)

Ellis, H. & Calne, R.Y. (1972)
Lecture Notes on General Surgery. Oxford: Blackwell.

Schwartz, S. (1975)
Principles of Surgery. New York: McGraw-Hill.

Index